STRUCTURED EXERCISES in WELLNESS PROMOTION

A WHOLE PERSON™ HANDBOOK FOR TRAINERS, EDUCATORS AND GROUP LEADERS

VOLUME I

edited by
Nancy Loving Tubesing, EdD
and
Donald A Tubesing, MDiv, PhD

Whole Person Press

Printed in the United States of America
by Port Cities Printing, Superior WI

10 9 8 7 6 5 4 3 2 1

Published by: **WHOLE PERSON PRESS**
PO Box 3151
Duluth MN 55803
218/728-4077

PREFACE

With the publication of this volume and its companion, <u>Structured Exercises in Stress Management Volume I</u>, we proudly inaugurate our new line of topical Whole Person Handbooks. Volume II in each series is scheduled for publication in January 1984.

The Whole Person Handbooks are specially designed for trainers, consultants, counselors, teachers, adult education specialists, nurses, psychologists, clergy, managers, group workers, health educators -- for anyone using the experiential approach to learning. Each Handbook contains a compilation of the best structured exercises for teaching wellness promotion or stress management, with complete instructions for your use. We've personally tested all of these processes in a variety of settings and believe that nowhere will you find a collection of more effective structured experiences for actively involving the participant -- as a whole person -- in the learning process.

As you will soon discover, many of these exercises we've designed ourselves and refined them in the more than 1,000 workshops we've conducted during the past 10 years. Some are new combinations of time-tested group process activities. Others were submitted by people like you who continually strive to add the creative touch in their teaching. Whenever we've been aware of the source of an idea, we've noted it.

Please note our policy for reproduction of the Handbook contents. Our purpose in publishing these volumes is to foster inter-professional networking and to provide a framework through which we can all share our most effective ideas with each other. The layout is designed for easy photocopying of worksheets and training notes.

In the Whole Person Handbook series we've shared our best with you and hope you'll return the favor. We encourage you to submit your favorite structured exercises for inclusion in future volumes. You'll find instructions in the contributor's section at the back of the book. Let us know what works well for you so that we can carry on the tradition of providing a forum for the exchange of innovative teaching designs.

Duluth MN
April 1983

Nancy Loving Tubesing
Donald A Tubesing

WHOLE PERSON ASSOCIATES INC

Whole Person Associates Inc, consultants and publishers, was created to fill a void in the professional continuing education and consultation arena. We specialize in designing workshops and innovative training materials on stress management, wellness promotion, burnout prevention, communication skills and related subjects.

Our unique interdisciplinary approach synthesizes theory and research, then integrates this knowledge with an educational process that attends to the whole person -- body, mind and spirit. Faculty Associates represent a variety of professional backgrounds including education, psychology, medicine, social work, nursing, counseling and ministry.

The bulk of our teaching activity is co-sponsored with community-based helping agencies, hospitals, mental health agencies, community colleges and governmental agencies, as well as with business and industry.

We would be pleased to discuss the possibility of scheduling an on-site workshop or consultation in your setting.

TABLE OF CONTENTS

ICEBREAKERS

WELLNESS

SELF-CARE

PLANNING

ENERGIZERS

INTRODUCTION

Wellness is the hot topic of the 80's. If you're prepared to
address the issue, you'll get plenty of opportunities. If you
creatively involve people in the learning process, your teaching
will be much more helpful than even the most entertaining lecture.

Effective teaching helps people move beyond information to imple-
mentation. Health education that really works involves people
in the process of reflecting, assessing, prioritizing, sorting,
planning for change and affirming progress.

Structured Exercises in Wellness Promotion Volume I offers you
36 designs you can use for getting people involved, whatever the
setting and time constraints, whatever the sophistication of the
audience. To aid you in the selection of appropriate exercises,
they are grouped into five broad categories:

> Icebreakers: These short (10-20 minutes) exercises are
> designed to introduce people to each other and to open
> up participants' thinking process regarding wellness.
> They are lively. All five engage people actively in the
> topic and with each other. Try combining an icebreaker
> with an exercise from the wellness or self-care section
> for an instant evening program.

> Wellness Exploration: These exercises explore the issue
> of wellness from the whole person perspective. Rather
> than focus merely on the physical, these five processes
> help people examine their overall lifestyle. You'll find
> a mixture of moderate length assessments (30-60 minutes)
> and major theme developers (60-120 minutes). Each exer-
> cise can easily be contracted or expanded to fit your
> purpose.

> Self-Care Strategies: The first two exercises engage
> participants in looking at self-care issues in general.
> The remaining nine focus on specific self-care strategies
> in six life dimensions: physical, emotional, mental,
> spiritual, relational and lifestyle well-being.

> Action Planning/Closure: These five exercises help
> participants draw together their insights and determine
> the actions they wish to take on their own behalf. Some
> of the activities also suggest rituals that bring closure
> to the group process.

> Energizers: The ten energizers are designed to perk up
> the group whenever fatigue sets in. Sprinkle them through-
> out your program as needed for a change of pace. Try one
> as an icebreaker. They're guaranteed to get everyone's
> juices (including yours!) flowing again in 5-10 minutes.

The Handbook format is designed for easy use. You'll find
that each exercise is described completely, including;

- goals
- group size
- time frame
- materials needed
- step-by-step process instructions
- variations

Special instructions to the trainer are typed in italics.
Scripts to be read to the group are typed in a sans serif face.
Questions to ask the group are preceded by a □。
Mini-lecture notes are preceded by a ● or a *.

The instructions are written primarily for large group (30-100
people) workshop settings, but most of the exercises work just
as well with small groups, in individual therapy and for personal reflection.

If you are teaching in the workshop or large group setting, we
believe that the use of small discussion groups is the most
potent learning structure available to you. We've found that
groups of four persons each provide ample "air time" and a good
variety of interaction. Let groups meet together two or three
different times before forming new groups.

These personal "sharing groups" allow people to make positive
contact with each other and encourage them to personalize their
experience in depth. On evaluations, some people will say,
"drop this," others will say, "give us more small group time,"
but most will report that the time you give them to share with
each other becomes the heart of the workshop.

If you are working with an intact group of 12 people or less,
you may at times want to keep the whole group together for
process and discussion time rather than divide into the sug-
gested four or six person groups.

Each trainer has personal strengths, biases, pet concepts and
processes. We expect and encourage you to expand and modify
what you find here to fit your style. Adjust the exercises as
you see fit. Bring these designs to life for your participants
by inserting your own content and examples into your teaching.
Experiment!

And when you come up with something new, let us know . . .

ICEBREAKERS

1. INTRODUCTIONS (p 1)

   This collection of brief get-acquainted exercises includes
   four creative processes for use at the beginning of a workshop or teaching session. (5-10 minutes)

2. TWO MINUTE MILL (p 5)

   Participants use the energy bond position and provocative
   questions to get acquainted with several other group
   members. (10-15 minutes)

3. HUMAN HEALTH/ILLNESS CONTINUUM (p 8)

   In this lively icebreaker participants physically place
   themselves in the room along a continuum representing
   current health status. (10-20 minutes)

4. BEAUTIFUL PEOPLE: A PINUP CONTEST (p 11)

   This icebreaker engages participants in creating a collage
   that portrays the advertising media's vision of how to be
   "super well." (10-20 minutes)

5. TEN QUALITIES OF THE "SUPER-WELL" (p 14)

   This short consensus-building exercise engages participants
   in an intense discussion of their concepts about health as
   well as their personal priorities and biases. (25-30 minutes)

1 INTRODUCTIONS

This collection of brief get-acquainted exercises includes four creative processes for use at the beginning of a workshop or teaching session.

GOALS

1) To provide a structure for participants to get acquainted.

2) To promote interaction among participants.

GROUP SIZE

Unlimited as long as the room has movable chairs and plenty of space for participants to spread out. Exercises may need to be adapted to fit a less flexible physical setting.

TIME FRAME

5-10 minutes

MATERIALS NEEDED

A blank sheet of paper for each participant.

PROCESS

ANALOGIES

Participants are asked to think about what health food they identify with most, then introduce themselves to the whole group by stating their name, the chosen health food and describing how they are like that particular food.

Note: The trainer may want to give an example such as: "I'm _____ and the food I chose was granola because I think of myself as having so many different textures and flavors, packed with energy, and a good companion not only in the morning, but throughout the day." Or, "I'm _____ and I chose salt substitute because I used to have high blood pressure and still watch my salt intake."

VARIATION

■ Instead of using the health food theme for analogies,

the participants could introduce themselves as a body part, as a health problem or disease, or as a specific remedy. If the group is larger than 15-20 people, this exercise will take more than 5-10 minutes and may get repetitious. The trainer could ask participants to form smaller groups (3-6 people) and introduce themselves.

AFFIRMATIONS

1) The trainer asks participants to jot down their answers to these four questions/unfinished statements -- noting that all change starts with self-acceptance:

   ☐ I am _____ ;

   ☐ Two things I really like about me _____
   _____ ;

   ☐ One thing I do well in my job _____
   *Note: The trainer may joke, "Your supervisor
   wouldn't have to agree with you!"*

   ☐ One thing I contribute to a loving, caring relationship _____ .

2) Participants are asked to introduce themselves to a neighbor, comparing answers to the first statement, then moving on to the next until both partners have shared all their affirmations.

VARIATION

■ The trainer may want to substitute affirmations tailored to the particular content of the session (e.g. "One way I take good care of myself . . .")

WELLNESS GOALS/HEALTH CONCERNS

1) The trainer asks participants to write down five or six health concerns. These may be major or minor pro-blems that they are currently experiencing. (2 minutes)

2) On another section of the paper, participants are asked to list several wellness goals that they hope to achieve. (2 minutes)

3) The trainer then asks participants to go back and

circle those goals and concerns they hope to work on
during this wellness promotion course or workshop.

4) Participants divide into groups of four and in turn
share whatever goals and concerns they wish with
others in the small group.

5) The large group is reconvened to move into the next
exercise.

VARIATIONS

■ Instead of dividing into groups of four, each participant could introduce herself to the whole group by
sharing, "One thing I'm hoping to work on during this
course . . ."

■ The trainer may want to expand this exercise into an
agenda-setting chalk talk by asking each small group to
identify seven goals and concerns they would like to
see addressed in the course. The group at large could
then discuss and prioritize the topics.

JINGLES

1) The trainer asks participants to think for a few
moments about a commercial jingle or advertisement
that in some way describes them (e.g. "You've come
a long way, baby," "Go for it," etc.)

2) Participants pair up and explain their choice of
jingles to their partners. (2 minutes)

3) The trainer asks each pair to join another pair
forming groups of four. Each person then introduces
his partner using the jingle.

VARIATIONS

■ In Step #3, participants could also be asked to
identify what health messages are implied by their
jingles. Other group members could help uncover the
hidden messages.

■ With groups over 25, instead of using advertising
slogans, the trainer could ask participants to choose
a family motto or adage to share with the group (e.g.
"Too many cooks spoil the broth"; "Pretty is as pretty
does").

TRAINER'S NOTES

"Affirmations" is the brainchild of Tom and Judy Wright,
Minneapolis, MN. "Wellness Goals/Health Concerns" is adapted
from The Wellness Kit, Aid Association for Lutherans,
Appleton WI.

2 TWO MINUTE MILL

Participants use the energy bond position and provocative questions to get acquainted with several other group members.

GOALS

1) To promote interaction among participants.

2) To raise issues related to the topic under study.

GROUP SIZE

Unlimited as long as the room has enough open space for participants to mill around freely.

TIME FRAME

10-15 minutes

PROCESS

1) The trainer asks participants to stand up, mill around in the large group, and choose someone as a partner.

2) Partners exchange names and then ask each other in turn the question: "What is one thing you want to learn today?" (1 minute)

3) The trainer calls time, then asks for a volunteer to help demonstrate the energy bond position:

The trainer and volunteer stand about two feet apart facing one another. Both people extend their hands in front of them with left palm up and right palm down, about midriff-high, until their palms touch lightly. The trainer's right hand will rest on the volunteer's upturned left hand. The volunteer's right hand rests palm down on the trainer's palm-up left hand.

4) After the demonstration, participants are directed to quickly find a new partner, assume the energy bond position, exchange names, then ask and answer the question: "What is one thing you want to learn today?" Once the pair has exchanged information, they disconnect, mill, find another partner, connect, share and move on. People will probably make 4-5 contacts in the 2 minute period.

5)   After 2 minutes the trainer calls time and poses a new
     question appropriate to the topic of the session.
     (See the "Provocative Questions" list for suggestions.)
     Participants continue to mill, connecting in the energy
     bond and sharing questions and answers with as many
     other people as possible during the 2 minutes.

6)   The exercise continues with a new question every 2
     minutes until the group seems fully energized and
     ready to tackle the next learning module.

7)   The trainer may want to solicit reactions and obser-
     vations from the group as large before moving on.

VARIATION

■ This lively exercise can be used anytime during a session
  to loosen up or energize the group.

TRAINER'S NOTES

Submitted by J J Cochran

PROVOCATIVE QUESTIONS

What's your most positive self-care trait?

What's your most pressing health-care concern?

What was the favorite remedy for sickness in your family?

What disease are you most afraid of getting?

What self-care habit would you most like to improve?

What's your most favorite and least favorite exercise?

What sports did you play as a child?

What's the most important part of your body to you?

What's one of your disabilities?

What are two of your most important values?

What brings you great joy?

When is the last time you cried?

What drugs do you keep in your desk/purse?

What food do you have a real weakness for?

What is the thing you most want in a friendship?

What is the most healthy relationship you have?

How much sleep is best for you?

When are you most likely to feel depressed?

What is the most important thing you own?

What is your normal resting pulse?

What's your favorite way to relax?

What's one thing you're truly committed to?

What's the last book you read that had an impact on you?

Who is one of your heroes/heroines?

What's the most important part of wellness?

How do you sabotage your self-care plans?

What do you do when you're bored?

How do you usually express your anger?

What's the most unhealthy aspect of your environment?

What's the healthiest aspect of your work situation?

When did you first have an alcoholic drink?

When did you have your first cigarette?

3 HUMAN HEALTH/ILLNESS CONTINUUM

In this lively icebreaker participants physically place themselves in the room along a continuum representing current health status. This process could be used as either an opening or closing exercise.

GOALS

1) To reveal underlying attitudes toward health.

2) To encourage interaction among participants.

GROUP SIZE

Unlimited; as long as the room has an area large enough for participants to place themselves on a line from one wall to the other; works best with 20 or more people.

TIME FRAME

Approximately 10-20 minutes.

PROCESS

1) The trainer asks participants to think for a moment about how they would judge their current state of health and to pay attention to the factors that influence their judgment.

2) The trainer designates a spot on one wall as "EXTREMELY HEALTHY, VITAL" and a spot on the opposite wall to represent "VERY POOR HEALTH."

   Participants are asked to imagine a line drawn on the floor connecting these points. This line becomes the health-illness continuum.

3) The trainer asks people to line up on the continuum, placing themselves according to how they perceive their current state of health.

   Note: The ambiguity of this task often causes anxiety. When participants ask for clarification, encourage them to place themselves according to their own perceptions, using whatever criteria they consider important.

4) Once participants are spread along the continuum the trainer may want to comment on the diversity or similarity in the group. Give some verbal support to those brave enough to admit that they have health problems; and congratulate those who are models of health.

5) The trainer then asks participants to find one or two others who are close by and discuss together the health factors that influenced their placement. What health problems moved them toward the illness end? What good habits or natural strengths moved them toward the health end?

6) Participants are asked to reflect on their health once again, this time trying to judge where others who know them well (e.g. their physician, spouse, parents or kids) might put them on the continuum.

7) The trainer asks people to move to the place where they think other people would place them on the continuum. (Some people may not need to move.)

8) Once everyone has moved the trainer may request a show of hands for those who: 1) moved toward health; 2) moved toward illness; 3) stayed the same.

9) Again participants find one or two others near them on the continuum and discuss together how significant people in their lives perceive their health and influence their self-care behaviors.

10) The trainer may reconvene the entire group and begin an in depth exploration of personal wellness styles.

VARIATIONS

■ After Step #5 or Step #9, the trainer may ask participants to rearrange themselves on the health/illness continuum according to one or more of these dimensions:

- mental health (self-concept, feelings, moods, creativity, curiosity)

- relational health (w/spouse, nuclear family, extended family, friends, social activity, outreach)

- spiritual health (sense of purpose, commitment, faith, values, hope, forgiveness)

- lifestyle health (stress management, consumption, spending patterns, conservation)

© 1983 Whole Person Press PO Box 3151 Duluth, MN 55803

- whole person (all dimensions)

■ If this process is used as a closing exercise, the trainer
  may ask participants to move to the point on the continuum
  where they would like to be three months from now.

  Then the trainer could ask them to identify three steps
  they are willing to take in the next month to move themselves toward that goal. Participants might share these
  goals with a neighbor on the continuum line.

TRAINER'S NOTES

4 BEAUTIFUL PEOPLE: A PIN UP CONTEST

This icebreaker engages participants in creating a collage that portrays the advertising media's vision of how to be "super well."

GOALS

1) To highlight the distorted images of health and false promises of wellness which bombard us through advertising.

2) To engage participants in a spirited, energizing activity.

GROUP SIZE

Any size is appropriate as long as the room is large enough for participants to spread out and move around freely.

TIME FRAME

10-20 minutes

MATERIALS NEEDED

One popular magazine for each participant; one piece of paper, posterboard or newsprint for each person; one roll of tape or bottle of glue for every 3-4 people; scissors are optional; blackboard.

PROCESS

1) The trainer gives each participant one piece of paper, newsprint or posterboard on which to form a collage. Each participant also receives one out-of-date mass circulation magazine. The trainer may ask participants to select one of their liking from a pile or a box.

2) The trainer instructs participants to page through the magazine and select one picture of a "beautiful person" who represents the look of true healthfulness. Each participant pastes this picture in the center of her collage as a "pin up." Participants give their "pin ups" a fictitious, but appropriate name -- the more humorous, the better!

3) Participants are then instructed to page through the
    magazine again, scanning the advertisements for messages
    that promise health and wellness through using a par-
    ticular product. Participants tear out pictures of
    such products, along with the phrases, slogans and
    words that seem to promote wellness. These clippings
    are then pasted around the "pin up" -- demonstrating
    the ways that this beautiful person can stay super
    well. (5-10 minutes)

    *Note: Encourage participants to be creative and
           humorous, placing remedies for headaches, and
           hemorrhoids, hernias and herpes, at "appropriate"
           locations in the collage.*

4) Participants then stand one-at-a-time, hold up their
    poster, introduce their "pin up" by name ("I'd like you
    to meet _____ "), and detail all the fine products
    this beautiful person must use to stay so vibrantly
    alive and beautiful. ("He stays attractive by applying
    _____ and by swallowing _____, and keeps many
    friends around by using _____ regularly.")

    *Note: * Encourage participants to make snide side com-
             ments and act out in any way they wish in
             order to elaborate the humor of the marketing
             promises pictured.*

           *   Keep the pace moving -- allowing only 30-40
               seconds for each poster.*

           *   If the group is large, the trainer may wish
               to divide the group into sections of 10-15
               persons each for this part of the exercise.*

5) The trainer points out that in reality the data on the
    poster regularly bombard our psyches, teaching us all
    the "tricks" for staying healthy. The trainer may ask,
    "What is it we learn?" and "How well does that learn-
    ing serve us?" The trainer leads the group in a
    short discussion of the issues highlighted by this
    experience, and may choose to list them on the black-
    board for future reference.

6) The posters/collages may be taped on the wall around
    the room as an additional demonstration of the bombard-
    ment we suffer and the messages that are subliminally
    etched onto our brains.

VARIATIONS

- An alternate poster session that makes a similar point could be called "Promises, "Promises, Promises . . ."

  Instead of selecting one "pin up" and many products to surround the "pin up" in Steps #2 and #3, participants could tear out and paste up several beautiful people, and then for each ad state the promised result of using the product. The trainer may want to give some examples of such implicit or explicit promises:

  - Marlboro Man cut out. "If you smoke Marlboros -- then you'll be rugged, and free, and get to ride horses in the mountains and wear sheepskin coats."

  - Black Velvet Bombshell cut out. "If you drink Black Velvet -- then you'll be smooth, sexy, and elegant."

  - Pepsi Generation cut out. "If you drink Pepsi -- you'll be a young, vibrant, beautiful person. Then you can play volleyball on the warm beach, in bikinis with other beautiful folks, and have the time of your life."

  Participants paste up as many beautiful people as they can in 6-8 minutes, and then write down all the subtle promises they see pictured in each ad. All other process instructions (Steps #4-6) remain the same as for Beautiful People.

TRAINER'S NOTES

5 TEN QUALITIES OF THE SUPER WELL

This short consensus-building exercise engages participants in an intense discussion of their concepts about health as well as their personal priorities and biases.

GOALS

1) To expand awareness of the various elements and complex issues that comprise the multi-dimensional subject of health.

2) To help participants discover their personal priorities concerning wellness.

GROUP SIZE

Any size group is appropriate.

TIME FRAME

25-30 minutes

MATERIALS NEEDED

"Ten Qualities of the Super-Well" worksheet for each participant; blackboard or newsprint easel.

PROCESS

1) The trainer supplies each participant with the worksheet listing qualities of health and wellness, then asks individuals to rank the listed items in order of importance. (5 minutes)

2) The participants are divided into groups of 6-8 persons and given 15 minutes to arrive at a group consensus on the ranking of the qualities of health.

Note: Consensus must be reached in a democratic fashion with each person's viewpoints taken seriously. Voting and tallying total points is not allowed. Consensus must be reached by discussion only!

3) Small groups report the results of their consensus to the total group. The trainer records each set of rankings on the board. Small group reporters are encouraged to explain their group's rationale for

controversial rankings.

4) The trainer asks for reactions and insights, and points out the wide variety of personal beliefs exhibited by the difference in rankings.

VARIATIONS

■ The trainer may wish to have the group brainstorm their own list of super-well qualities, then rank that list, rather than utilizing the items on the worksheet.

■ If time is limited, Step #2 could be dropped, with individuals reporting their top three qualities to the group at large.

■ The "Ten Qualities of the Super-Well" could be used in conjunction with Exercise #9 as the subject of a Wellness Congress.

TRAINER'S NOTES

TEN QUALITIES OF THE SUPER-WELL
WORKSHEET

Rank the 10 items in order of importance as you judge them . . .
(most important = 1; least important = 10)

To be super-well one needs to be:

_____ Deeply committed to a cause outside oneself.

_____ Physically able to do whatever one wants with intensity
        and great energy -- seldom sick.

_____ A caring and loving person on whom others lean in a crisis.

_____ In tune with the spiritual -- having a clear sense of
        purpose and direction.

_____ Intellectually sharp, able to handle information; posses-
        sing an ever-curious mind and a good sense of humor.

_____ Well-organized and able to accomplish great quantities of
        work.

_____ Able to live in and enjoy the present, rather than focus-
        ing on the past or looking toward the future.

_____ Comfortable with experiencing the full range of human
        emotions.

_____ Accepting of one's limitations, handicaps and mistakes.

_____ Able and willing to take charge of one's life, to prac-
        tice positive self-care and to be assertive when
        necessary.

WELLNESS

6. WHOLE PERSON HEALTH APPRAISAL (p 17)

   In this novel health appraisal process participants draw
   on their own wisdom to assess their level of physical,
   mental, emotional, social, spiritual and lifestyle health.
   (20-30 minutes)

7. FOUR CORNERS (p 23)

   In this reflection-action exercise, participants fantasize
   the long-run implication of their whole person self-care
   habits and lifestyle choices by imagining what type of
   health breakdown they are headed toward. (15-20 minutes)

8. VITALITY FACTORS (p 25)

   This exercise allows individuals to assess their strengths
   and weaknesses in unique areas of high vitality (e.g.
   body maintenance, letting go, celebrating, etc.).
   (30-45 minutes)

9. WELLNESS CONGRESS (p 30)

   This exercise opens up for participants the wide range of
   issues and factors to be considered as part of health and
   wellness by challenging them to formulate and adopt a
   group creed of wellness. (90-120 minutes)

10. HEALTH/ILLNESS IMAGES (p 37)

    This extended reflection exercise helps participants
    recognize the ebb and flow of sickness and health in their
    lives, and uncover personal symbols that shape their life-
    style patterns. (90 minutes)

6 WHOLE PERSON HEALTH APPRAISAL

In this novel health appraisal process participants draw on their own wisdom to assess their level of physical, mental, emotional, social, spiritual and lifestyle health. Participants then identify their personal health risk areas.

GOALS

1) To raise participants' consciousness about the many aspects of health.

2) To appraise personal well-being from a whole person perspective.

3) To identify personal health risk factors in a variety of life dimensions.

GROUP SIZE

Unlimited; also appropriate for work with individuals.

TIME FRAME

20-30 minutes

MATERIALS NEEDED

"Whole Person Health Appraisal" and "Risk Factors" worksheets for each participant.

PROCESS

1) The trainer introduces the concept of health appraisals and risk factors, describing the traditional health risk appraisal and contrasting the whole person appraisal process. During this chalk talk, the trainer may want to include some or all of these ideas:

- The traditional health risk appraisal focuses specifically on areas of health and risk where researchers can provide quantifiable data.

- Such appraisals rely on statistical correlations between death rates (or illness/accident incidence) and quantifiable physical qualities and habits.

- The whole person appraisal offers another way to view health and risk factors. This appraisal taps in to the internal wisdom of the individual rather than external data and focuses on all dimensions of well-being (including mental, emotional, social, spiritual and lifestyle issues), rather than primarily the physical.

- Both types of appraisal provide feedback regarding personal risk factors as well as recommended actions a person can adopt to increase the probability of a longer, more satisfying life.

2) The trainer distributes the "Whole Person Appraisal" worksheets and instructs participants to first consider their physical health, circling items in the physical portion of the appraisal which may give them trouble and starring items that signal wellness. The trainer encourages people to add any additional qualities or attributes that occur to them.

3) The trainer then leads the participants through the other five dimensions of the health assessment, describing each as he goes along and allowing time for the circling and starring of appropriate items.

4) When everyone is finished, the trainer asks participants to reflect on the quality of their health in each separate dimension and to fill in the thermometer for each dimension, according to their judgment of their current health status in that area. After participants have completed the mental, emotional, social, spiritual and lifestyle thermometers, they will have an overall picture of their whole person wellness in thermometer form.

5) The trainer distributes the "Risk Factor" worksheet to participants and directs them to focus on potential risk factors in each dimension of well-being. Each person should identify one or more personal attitudes or habits in each dimension that increase his risk of future dis-ease.

   Note: A "Risk Factor" is defined as any attribute, attitude, habit or behavior pattern that, if continued, is likely to cause problems and decrease the quality of life in the future.

6) Each participant finds a partner who will act as his "personal consultant." Each pair decides who will act as consultant first. The other partner acts first as client.

7) The client is given five minutes to describe his appraisal to his consultant and to target two or three risk factors he would like to change. The consultant

is then given five minutes to interview the client
further, helping him formulate a plan of action that
will reduce these risk factors.

8) The partners switch roles (client becomes consultant)
and repeat Steps #6 and #7.

VARIATIONS

■ Some trainers may want to use this whole person appraisal
process in tandem with a more traditional health risk
appraisal to help participants get a better picture of
overall health concerns and to increase their motivation
for change.

■ Steps #6-8 may be completed in small groups, with each
member taking a turn as "client" while the rest of the
group acts as "consultants."

■ Participants could draw their thermometers (Step #4) on
newsprint posters and hang them around the room. This
would be particularly effective as the "before" picture
at the beginning of a several week course. At the closing
session, participants could make an "after" poster thermometer, showing the changes they have made during the inter-
vening weeks.

TRAINER'S NOTES

WHOLE PERSON HEALTH APPRAISAL

Circle the items with which you are not satisfied at present.
** Star the items that signal your wellness.

PHYSICAL			
smoking	caffeine intake	alcohol use	medications
weight	physical pain	sexual satisfaction	exercise
energy	body tension	body image	other
stamina	sleep patterns	diet habits	
strength	general health	attention I pay to my body	

MENTAL			
alertness	poetic vision	memory	enthusiasm
creativity	know my field	wise	stimulating
new ideas	open-minded	capable	other
logical	consistent	curiosity	

EMOTIONAL			
depressed	often anxious	can express feelings	happy
stability	often scared	can accept feelings	other
sensitive	self-confidence	meet my own needs	
grieving	feel secure	in touch with me	
freedom	self-control	sense of success	
content	independence	all together	

SOCIAL			
friendship	handle conflict	meet all people w/ ease	affectionate
intimacy	social graces	express needs to others	polite
outgoing	conversation ease	respond to others' needs	entertaining
respect	able to say "no"	relationship w/ spouse	other
honesty	loyal -- trusting	relationship w/ kids	
obedient	am helpful	relationship w/ parents	
tolerant	forgiveness	dependent/independent	

THERMOMETER OF
MY STATE OF HEALTH

Physical
Mental
Emotional
Social
Spiritual
Life Style

Perfect

Excellent

Adequate

Room for
Improvement

Holds Me Back

Poor

Critical

Fill Mercury
up to
Appropiate Level

SPIRITUAL

hope
meaning
purpose
values
faith

positive view
feel forgiven
good example
worship life
at peace

comfort w/ my death
worthwhileness
in touch w/ God
sharing faith
prayer life

commitment
direction
submission
other

LIFE STYLE

habits
priorities
courageous
satisfied
orderliness

moved recently
going too fast
trying too hard
able to relax
able to enjoy

comfortable w/ aging
handle money well
appreciate beauty
job satisfaction
desision-making

able to play
goal setting
successful
other

MY PERSONAL RISK FACTORS

What factors in your current health picture and self-care patterns are presently causing difficulty in your life or are
likely to cause you some problems in the future? What patterns,
if continued, will diminish the quality of your life one year
from now? Ten years from now?

Physical

Mental

Emotional

Social

Spiritual

Lifestyle

7 FOUR CORNERS

In this reflection-action exercise, participants fantasize
the long-run implication of their whole person self-care
habits and lifestyle choices by imagining what type of
health breakdown they are headed toward. This exercise is
most effective when preceded by some form of whole person
health habit assessment.

GOALS

1) To identify the long-run consequences of whole person
    health habits and lifestyle choices.

2) To explore strategies for preventing health breakdown.

3) To energize the group and promote interaction.

GROUP SIZE

Any size as long as the room has adequate space for group
members to gather in the four corners; some modification
necessary for groups smaller than 12.

TIME FRAME

15-20 minutes

PROCESS

1) The trainer introduces the concept that our negative
    health habits and lifestyle choices in all dimensions
    of life, if continued over time, will eventually
    result in a health breakdown. The trainer will need
    to describe the four areas of potential health break-
    down.

    • Those people with poor physical self-care patterns
      are most likely headed for some sort of physical
      illness.

    • People who neglect or abuse their relationships
      may find themselves in hot water with family mem-
      bers or without a friend in the world.

    • Too much stimulation and change can lead to mental
      fatigue or emotional upheaval; too little is a set-
      up for boredom, stagnation and depression.

    • Poor spiritual self-care habits -- lack of purpose,

cynicism, half-hearted commitments -- ultimately result in emptiness, despair and crises of doubt.

2) The trainer asks participants to reflect on their self-care patterns in the four dimensions of life (physical, mental, relational, spiritual) and decide, based on their present lifestyle and health habits, what type of health breakdown they are working toward.

3) The trainer designates the four corners of the room:

   ☐ "the physical illness or accident ward"
   ☐ "the mental fatigue or emotional upheaval unit"
   ☐ "the relationship difficulties and lonely hearts corral"
   ☐ "the spiritual emptiness pit"

Participants are instructed to move to the treatment corner they are most likely to need if they continue their current patterns.

4) Once participants are gathered in their corners, the trainer asks them to pair up with one or two others and discuss together the specific habits and patterns that put them in this corner. (5-7 minutes)

5) Staying in the same small groups, participants are then asked to identify some ways they could prevent this health breakdown from occurring.

TRAINER'S NOTES

8 VITALITY FACTORS

This exercise allows individuals to assess their strengths and weaknesses in unique areas of high vitality (e.g. body maintenance, letting go, celebrating, etc). Participants make specific commitments to modify and improve their life-style. This exercise is excellent for structuring between-session homework or post-workshop follow-up.

GOALS

1) To identify personal vitality factors.

2) To identify areas for revitalization.

3) To provide structure and motivation for lifestyle changes.

GROUP SIZE

Any size; also appropriate for work with individuals.

TIME FRAME

Chalk talk 20-30 minutes; assessment 10-15 minutes.

MATERIALS NEEDED

Chalk board or newsprint easel; "Vitality Analysis and Action Form" for all participants.

PROCESS

1) The trainer introduces the concept of high vitality as a component of wellness and chooses 6-12 vitality factors to outline for the group. The trainer focuses on factors particularly appropriate to the training group or chooses some from the list below.
    * nutrition practices
    * physical fitness
    * getting and giving positive strokes
    * keeping in touch with youth
    * managing change in your life
    * working hard
    * getting away from work
    * growth and stimulation
    * optimistic attitude
    * consistency, dependability, commitment
    * interesting friends and colleagues

* sense of humor
* enthusiasm
* support systems
* guiding philosophy of life
* celebration
* letting go

Each vitality factor should have a concise and descrip-
tive name that is written on the chalkboard or newsprint as it is explained in detail.

2) The trainer asks participants to rank the vitality
    factors in order of their present levels of competence
    in each, putting the factor that is most active in
    their life at the top and the factor that is least
    utilized at the bottom.

3) The trainer distributes the "Vitality Assessment and
    Action Form" and asks participants to choose two
    vitality factors for special attention, writing one
    factor at the top of the left worksheet and one at the
    top of the right worksheet.

    *Note: Some people may choose to focus on a vitality
            factor at which they already feel competent.
            Fine. Encourage those folks to affirm their
            strength and apply it even more effectively.*

4) Using the worksheet, participants are asked to focus
    on one factor at a time, assessing their present
    level of competence, desired level of competence, cur-
    rent evidence of competence and areas for growth to
    improve the vitality factor. At the bottom, partici-
    pants list specific steps they are willing to take in
    order to move toward a higher vitality level, along
    with a specific date for implementation of each
    strategy.

5) The trainer may ask for volunteers to publicly affirm
    their commitments to high vitality by reading the list
    of actions they plan to undertake.

    *Note: If this exercise is being used for homework
            between sessions, be sure participants choose
            at least one or two strategies that can be
            implemented in the intervening time. At the
            beginning of the next session the trainer can
            ask for "success stories" to be shared with the
            group.*

    If this exercise is used as part of a workshop

*or as a closing planning process, the trainer
may want to collect the forms and mail them to
participants 3-6 months later.*

VARIATIONS

■ Instead of presenting a predetermined list of vitality
factors, the trainer could ask the group to brainstorm
their own list. To stimulate this process, participants
could be asked to think about the most lively, vital person they know and then list the qualities that contribute
to that person's vitality.

Once a list is on the board, the trainer could choose
6-12 factors for further expansion and ranking, or allow
participants to choose from the larger list.

■ Between Step #2 and Step #3 the group could be divided
into smaller consultant groups. The trainer would post
newsprint pages around the room, each with a different
vitality factor written at the top. All those who ranked
a particular factor at the top of their list (highly com-
petent) would be designated as "visiting experts" on that
vitality factor and move to the newsprint poster for that
factor. (Everyone is an "expert" at some factor!) Once
all have moved to their consultation spot, the group
gathered at each poster spends 3-5 minutes brainstorming
ideas about how anyone could increase vitality in this
area of life. Creativity and humor are are encouraged!

Continue with Step #3. As part of Step #4, participants
could be given time to wander around the room, find the
posters for the vitality factors they have chosen to
improve, and write down all the suggestions they want to
remember from the "panel of experts."

TRAINER'S NOTES

Submitted by Tom Boman

VITALITY ANALYSIS AND ACTION FORM

Vitality Factor _____

PRESENT Level of Competence (Where I think I am)

1	2	3	4	5	6	7	8	9	10

Low   High

DESIRED Level of Competence (Where I'd like to be)

1	2	3	4	5	6	7	8	9	10

Low   High

Areas of Competence (What I know and do to achieve the vitality
                     factor):

Areas for Growth (What I need to learn and do to improve my
                  vitality factor):

Things I will start doing to improve my vitality factor:

        What (list)   When (now? this week? in 6
                                      months? sometime?)

1.

2.

3.

4.

Signature_____   _____
                                   (date of analysis)

VITALITY ANALYSIS AND ACTION FORM

Vitality Factor _____

PRESENT Level of Competence (Where I think I am)

1	2	3	4	5	6	7	8	9	10

Low   High

DESIRED Level of Competence   (Where I'd like to be)

1	2	3	4	5	6	7	8	9	10

Low   High

<u>Areas of Competence</u>   (What I know and do to achieve the vitality
                       factor):

<u>Areas for Growth</u>   (What I need to learn and do to improve my
                       vitality factor):

<u>Things I will start doing to improve my vitality factor:</u>

       <u>What</u> (list)   <u>When</u> (now? this week? in 6
                                         months? sometime?

  1.

  2.

  3.

  4.

Signature _____   _____
                                   (date of analysis)

© 1983 Whole Person Press   PO Box 3151   Duluth, MN 55803

9 WELLNESS CONGRESS

This exercise opens up for participants the wide range of issues and factors to be considered as part of health and wellness, by asking them to examine their own beliefs, and by challenging them as a total group to formulate and adopt a group creed of wellness.

GOALS

1) To help participants recognize their own beliefs and biases.

2) To stimulate spirited discussion regarding the qualities of whole person health and their relative importance.

3) To engage the group in a consensus building process.

GROUP SIZE

Any size is appropriate as long as the setting allows for small caucus groups as well as a plenary congressional session with representatives meeting in the center of the room.

TIME FRAME

90-120 minutes

MATERIALS NEEDED

Blank paper for all participants; a copy of the "Wellness Congress Caucus Instructions" for each caucus group; "Universal Congress on Wellness Session I Instructions"; blackboard or newsprint board.

PROCESS

1) The trainer describes the nature of a creed and outlines the task challenging the group. The trainer will want to include some or all of these points.

    ● Every person holds a unique collection of personal beliefs -- no two people ever believe exactly the same thing.

    ● Creeds are statements by a group of people regarding the beliefs they hold in common.

- Creeds are official public affirmations that each member of the group adheres to.

- In the history of religion many conferences with hundreds of participants have spent countless days trying to formulate creedal statements that capture the shared beliefs exactly. Sometimes consensus was never reached, and church groups split up, or wars were fought over the differences.

2) The trainer asks each participant individually to examine his beliefs about wellness. The trainer reads the following phrases one at a time and asks participants to write down as many answers as they can for each. (10 minutes)

    ☐ I believe wellness is . . .
    ☐ A person who is healthy . . .
    ☐ You regain and maintain full health by . . .
    ☐ When you're not well you're . . .
    ☐ Wellness includes all aspects of life such as . . .

Note: These questions can be asked one at a time, or a worksheet may be provided.

The trainer then asks participants independently to look over their sentence completions and write a summary paragraph that captures their beliefs about wellness.

3) The trainer divides the participants into smaller caucus groups of five to ten persons and gives a copy of the "Wellness Congress Caucus Instructions" to each group. The caucus groups draw up their wellness creeds. (15 minutes)

Note: For successful completion of Step #4, "The Congress," the trainer will want to create 6-12 caucus groups.

4) Chairs are placed in the center of the room and each caucus group sends one representative to the Universal Congress on Wellness.

Note: If there are only 2-5 caucus groups, then allow 2 or 3 representatives per group.

The trainer gives each representative a copy of the "Universal Congress on Wellness Session I Instructions" and clarifies any questions from the group. The

trainer sets a time limit for the session. Two
minutes times the number of representatives works well.

5) Exactly at the conclusion of the designated time a
    recess is called and representatives return to their
    caucus groups for 10 minutes of discussion.

    The caucus groups should be informed that Session 2
    of the congress will be the final meeting, and that
    by the end of the session the representatives must
    have drafted a creed to which all participants can
    ascribe.

6) At the conclusion of the recess the trainer reconvenes
    the representatives for the final 20 minute session of
    the Universal Congress on Wellness. The trainer
    reiterates that within 20 minutes the representatives
    must have completed the group's wellness creed.

    *Note: Be sure that at the conclusion of the congress
    a written creed is in clear public display for
    all participants to see*

    *If time is available, the trainer may choose to
    allow for three sessions of the congress, rather
    than two.*

7) The trainer asks participants to reflect individually
    on the creed that has been adopted. (10 minutes)

    The following questions may be raised by the trainer:

    □ On a scale of 0-10 how accurately does the group
      creed reflect your own beliefs? (0="not at all,"
      10="totally reflects my beliefs")

    □ Which statements do you disagree with? Which
      beliefs of yours are not included?

    □ Based on this creed would you be comfortable
      joining this group? Why? Why not?

    □ How well do you think the representatives compro-
      mised? What is the result and the cost of this
      compromise? Is the creed inclusive (whole person)
      or exclusive (only touching areas of wellness that
      match the group's biases)?

8) Participants return to their caucus groups and share
    their answers to these questions and any leftover
    reactions raised by the process. (10-20 minutes)

9) The trainer reconvenes the total group and asks for
    reactions and feedback, being sure to highlight the
    varieties of approaches to wellness and the major
    issues that surfaced. (10-20 minutes)

VARIATIONS

■ For groups of 15 or less, eliminate the caucus divisions
  and keep all participants together in one group for the
  Congress assembly.

■ If time is limited, Steps #4-6, "The Universal Congress
  on Wellness," may be eliminated. All other steps remain
  the same. The issues would then be dealt with only in
  the smaller caucus groups with individuals judging how
  well their personal beliefs fit in with the consensus
  statement of their caucus group. (Step #8)

  Cancellation of the Congress would save 45-50 minutes,
  but would also eliminate the opportunity for total
  group interaction and team-building.

■ Prior to the Congress (Step #4) the trainer could choose
  to assign 3-5 persons the role of viewing the entire
  proceedings as "critics-at-large."

  These critics could be empowered with one of the following
  three charges:

  a) To watch as if they were citizens of another culture,
      and focus their comments as if they were foreigners
      not familiar with the beliefs and assumptions of our
      culture.

  b) To assess and comment on the process of group inter-
      action as it unfolds in the caucus groups and the
      Universal Congress proceedings.

      ● Did everyone's ideas get considered?
      ● Did splinter groups want to pull out of the
          congress?
      ● Were any "holy" wars started by disagreements on
          orthodoxy?

  c) To judge the quality of the creed adopted by the
      Universal Congress according to all or some of the
      following nine yardsticks: (A worksheet checklist
      may be produced to facilitate this process.)

      Does the creed . . .

      ● include a focus on quality of life as well as
          quantity?

- acknowledge that health is a process not a goal?

- acknowledge and embrace death as a part of life?

- look beyond the body to include all elements of life?

- make provisions for personal limitations and handicaps whether physical, relational, spiritual, etc.?

- activate the forgiveness factor, by allowing people to deal with imperfection and short comings?

- acknowledge that high level wellness implies a connection to powers and purposes bigger than and beyond the individual?

- clearly indicate that personal responsibility and active self-care is essential in the development of wellness?

- challenge people to be "well-to-do . . ." and to be committed to caring for others and making a positive difference in their world as a result of their personal wellness?

The critics-at-large may be asked to report their observations immediately after the conclusion of the Universal Congress (Step #6) -- or as part of the closing discussion in Step #9.

TRAINER'S NOTES

WELLNESS CONGRESS CAUCUS
INSTRUCTIONS

1) You have 15 minutes to complete this task.

2) If you don't already know one another, introduce yourselves.

3) Each group member in turn should read her answers to the belief statements and her summary paragraph about wellness beliefs.

4) After everyone's individual beliefs have been heard the caucus group should formulate a tentative written "creed of wellness" that incorporates all issues raised. The group must reach a consensus, with every member agreeing with the caucus group's draft position statement.

5) Select one representative (or more, if directed by the trainer) to present your creed to the Universal Congress on Wellness.

6) All other caucus members will act as observers at the Congress.

**UNIVERSAL CONGRESS ON WELLNESS
SESSION I INSTRUCTIONS**

1) Each representative should present his caucus group's
   position statement to the congress. (1 minute each)

2) After everyone has been heard, all representatives work
   together to create a creedal statement on wellness that
   includes the major issues presented. The trainer will
   give you a time limit. At the end of this period there
   will be a 10 minute recess for consultation with your
   caucus groups before the congress reconvenes its final
   session.

3) Follow these guidelines in your deliberations:

   a) Only representatives are allowed to speak. Caucus
      members should listen closely to the discussion,
      but remain silent.

   b) You are allowed to appoint a recorder to keep track
      of major issues on the blackboard or newsprint.

   c) Caucus group members should note strategies they
      wish to suggest to their representative at the
      recess.

10 HEALTH/ILLNESS IMAGES

This extended reflection exercise helps participants
recognize the ebb and flow of sickness and health in their
lives, and uncover personal symbols that shape their lifestyle patterns. The four segments include a chalk talk,
guided reflection, small group sharing and plenary discussion of insights.

GOALS

1) To help participants recognize the patterns of health
   and illness they exhibit over their lifetime.

2) To help participants identify the major symbols and
   life scripts that drive their lifestyle decision-
   making.

3) To foster more conscious decision-making for self-care
   among participants.

GROUP SIZE

Any size group is appropriate. The power of this exercise
depends on three factors: an atmosphere of exploration
fostered by the trainer, the individual's discovery through
reflection and the personal sharing in small groups.

TIME FRAME

90 minutes

MATERIALS NEEDED

Blank sheets of paper for each participant.

PROCESS

Note: This exercise will be most effective when preceded
       by an exploration of personal health habits and when
       supported by an emphasis on personal responsibility
       for practicing positive self-care.

       The process outlined in the health/illness images
       is primarily reflective in nature and cannot be
       hurried. This exercise is not appropriate for
       situations where conceptual content and a lecture
       style are expected.

1) The trainer opens the session with a short warm-up chalk talk which introduces the subject of personal lifestyle choices and the major health/illness patterns that result. (5-10 minutes)

   Note: *See the Health/Illness Images Script, Part A (pp 41-42), for specific chalk talk notes.*

   The purpose of this lecturette is to create an atmosphere of reflection in which participants are invited to explore their intuitive mind and to discover the underlying symbols that unify the individual health/illness events of their lives which usually seem so discrete and disconnected.

   It is essential that the trainer slow down her pace in the opening talk to set the tone for the reflection which follows.

2) The trainer reads the Health/Illness questions provided in Part B of the script (pp 42-47) and asks participants to write down their answers. (25-30 minutes)

   Note: *The questions should be asked one by one, at a slow pace that allows ample time for reflection. No worksheet is provided, since this exercise is more effective if participants focus on only one question at a time, without knowing what comes next. Participants write their notes on blank paper distributed by the trainer.*

   Occasionally a few participants will be puzzled by a particular question. It is not necessary to "force" insights. Encourage them to simply wait for the next question which they will undoubtedly find more meaningful.

3) The trainer divides the participants into small groups or utilizes previously formed sharing groups of four persons each. Group members, one at a time, take five minutes to share whatever they wish regarding their answers to the questions and the ideas and insights that occurred to them as they wrote their responses. (25-30 minutes)

   Note: *The trainer may want to suggest that participants begin their sharing by showing the group the two pictures they drew of themselves, then proceed to sharing whatever else they wish.*

After each participant has had five minutes to share, the trainer directs the small groups to continue their discussion, focusing on the similarities and differences they discovered in each other's patterns of health/illness. (5-10 minutes)

4) The trainer reconvenes the group for plenary discussion of insights and observations. The trainer may wish to raise some or all of the following theme questions during the discussion:

□ What did you find when you compared your summary word for illness and your summary word for health?

Are they on the same continuum? Are they positive traits overdone? Ask for some examples of word pairs from the group.

□ Ask people what they found when they compared their pictures of themselves being sick and being well.

Often people find that the sickness picture had no face and no other people around, but the wellness picture had a face and other people in it. Ask for comments on any surprises.

□ Ask for the attitudes about sickness that people uncovered.

Some people demonstrate a "chicken soup" attitude toward sickness. For them, sickness means, "Whew!, Finally I can have an excuse to stop working and let other people help take care of me!"

Other people experience an anger reaction to sickness and they talk back to their bodies by saying, "No, you can't be sick today. Look at all the things on my list that I have to do!"

Of course, the body ends up using its veto power at some point if it's not responded to.

□ Help people see that wellness and sickness are not incompatible.

Most of us have enough sickness symptoms at all times to call ourselves sick if we want to. Most of us also have enough wellness symptoms all the time to label ourselves well if we so choose. You can be well and still have imperfections. You can be sick and still have various levels of wellness in your life.

□ Ask people to notice how they choose and manipulate their symptoms.

For example, a rural Minnesota road grader operator
confessed, "My daughter knows that if she's worried or
discouraged, she must still go to school, but if she
has a temperature, she doesn't have to. She can raise
her temperature anytime she wants to. You know how I
know that for sure? . . . I used to do it to my mother!"

☐ Reiterate again that wellness and sickness are to some
extent the result to the daily choices we make to do
small favors or disfavors for ourselves. Some of our
health, perhaps a sizable portion, relates directly to
our lifestyle choices.

☐ The trainer may want to caution against pushing the
idea of personal responsibility too far. There is no
scientific evidence that the individual who suffers
from cancer personally and consciously chose that
disease.

Note: *These and many other themes and issues will
probably arise spontaneously from the group.
The trainer needn't lecture or feel compelled
to cover them all. Be flexible and have fun
with whatever points the group brings up.*

TRAINER'S NOTES

HEALTH/ILLNESS IMAGES SCRIPT

A. WARM-UP CHALK TALK SCRIPT

- Just as a wind on the water produces both fleeting ripples which calm quickly, and great swells which slowly rise and fall in rhythm over the ages -- so also by our minor decisions hour by hour we engage in daily microscopic units of health/illness behavior that produce the deeper undulating patterns of our life. These add a wider context of ebb and flow to our years.

- Illness results not from a single destructive behavior, but from imbalance in this ebb and flow. Conversely wellness results from a wide pattern of health enhancing behaviors, not from a single solution applied once. We tend by our choices to get ourselves sick in the same old way over and over again; and we tend to help ourselves seek wellness and get better through activation of oft-repeated personal health patterns to which we return whenever illness forces us to adjust.

- These patterns are activated by personal symbols locked deep within our bosom. Seldom does our conscious mind catch a glimpse of these shadowy forms in which our decisions are rooted. Nevertheless with heavy handed guidance they shape our every behavior.

- What does the ebb and flow of sickness and health in your life look like, and what are the personal symbols that shape these patterns for you?

- The series of questions which follow are designed to help you discover the illness and the wellness rhythms below the surface of your life.

- Some questions will produce sparks of insight for you, others won't and that's OK. Play with your reactions. Go with the 5% of your mind that spits up impulse answers and see where they take you as you follow. Try not to be too rational. Your best responses will be illogical. After all -- you're trying to discover symbols and images in the recesses of your mind, not think logically in the same old way.

  Please take out a blank sheet of paper. First I'll ask you some questions that get at your illness style, then some that focus on your wellness style. Finally, I'll ask you to compare and contrast your two styles.

OK. Here we go. Just sit back and let your mind wander
as you write your reflections on the questions.

B. THE HEALTH/ILLNESS QUESTIONS SCRIPT

Sickness Style

1) Recall the last three times you were sick (under the
   weather).

   Note: *This is the key question in the sickness ser-*
   ies. Massage it a bit, after people have a
   minute to think, answer the puzzled looks by
   helping people broaden their idea of sickness
   (e.g. no good ideas for three months = sick,
   depressed and irritable may be sick).

   Give people time here. If they don't answer
   this, they won't get much out of the other
   questions.

2) Make some notes to yourself about what was going on
   in your life at each of those times. Don't write a
   paragraph, but just surround each of those occasions
   with some words.

   Questions like: What were you trying to accomplish?
   How were you feeling about work? What were some of
   the pressures there? Who were you living with? Where
   were you living? How were you feeling about yourself?
   What had you been engaged in? What were you looking
   forward to in the future?

   Make some notes to yourself about the dynamics and
   the tone of your life at each of those times when you
   got sick.

   Note: *Again, this is an important question. People*
   must get far enough into the mood to see some
   patterns. The questions which follow about
   style are milked from the answers here. Be sure
   to give enough good examples yourself, and to
   allow plenty of time for people to think.

3) Make a statement on your illness style as seen in
   these three sickness occasions. For example, "From

what I see here, my style of illness is <u>I go too fast and finally fall apart</u>."

4) Summarize that sickness style in one word that catches the feeling tone of that style -- one word that catches the flavor.

5) Draw a picture of yourself with your illness in it.

> *Note:* You might want to give people an example of your own on the blackboard and then tell them that they can draw a picture at least as good as yours. Be sure to have them both draw the picture and show their illness in it. You might need to encourage people just to get their pencils moving, even if they don't know how they want to draw themselves. Watch the group, some smiles and some sharing will start to occur.

6) Exaggerate the illness until you die of it. What do you die of?

> *Note:* When giving examples, don't give examples of "real" diseases. Try to show people that they can make up their own new diseases (e.g. "I get so tight around my shoulders that I suffocate myself"). You might tell people that the "disease" does not have to be found in the International Disease Classification Index.

7) Flip the sentence over so that your disease is an action that you are engaging in. For example, instead of saying, "I die of suffocation," say "I am suffocating myself." Instead of saying, "I die of a broken back," say "I am breaking my back." Write the statement that claims you are dis-easing yourself. See how that feels.

8) If you had to give up this illness and couldn't have it anymore, what else would you lose, what else would you have to give up?

9) What does that mean that you are, therefore, getting out of your disease?

10) Is that something you're willing to give up? Don't be too quick to answer. Probably you haven't been willing to give up this gain as of yet. Perhaps, your sickness is a small price to pay for what you're getting out of it.

> *Note:* *After asking these three questions, you might*
> *point out to people that these three are ques-*
> *tions regarding secondary gains. None of us*
> *would continue to engage in negative patterns*
> *unless they gave us something positive as well.*
> *These questions are very useful when trying to*
> *help somebody who obviously desires to change*
> *but has not yet been able to make the changes.*
> *Helping people see what they're getting out of*
> *their negative pattern gives them the opportunity*
> *to make a clearer choice, or to test out whether*
> *they can find another way to get what they want*
> *without creating the negative results.*

11) When do you plan the next episode of this disease?
    After you laugh, put down a date.

12) Now that you have thought about it, do you plan to go
    through with that appointment? Or, would you like to
    move it up a week so that you can do it on company
    time, or move it back a week so that it's more con-
    venient?

> *Note:* *In the Wholistic Health Centers we used to ask*
> *people this question. We offered to make an*
> *appointment for before their illness, during*
> *their illness, or right after their illness.*
> *Give an example or two about how people mani-*
> *pulate their illnesses (e.g. "I have been sick*
> *30 out of 37 Thanksgivings in my life. Either*
> *that means there's a powerful Thanksgiving Day*
> *virus that I'm allergic to, or it means I'm*
> *consistently doing something in my life pattern*
> *that helps me fall apart at that point in the*
> *fall when I give myself permission to do so").*
> *A woman recently said, "My kid said to me, 'Mom,*
> *please don't get sick this Christmas.'" We*
> *asked her, "What did you do?" She answered,*
> *"I waited until after New Year's."*
>
> *Be sure and ask people what they would have to*
> *change in order to manipulate the date forward*
> *or back.*

13) What's the message that you're broadcasting to the
    world about your beliefs by your sickness style? You
    are making a non-verbal assertion to the world about
    your beliefs by the way you are living your life and
    by your patterns for getting yourself sick. What is
    the belief that you're broadcasting?

Note: *This question is sometimes difficult for people.*
Give an example (e.g. "My belief is that I have
to do it by myself and prove my worth by what
kinds of work I get done. I feel more worth-
while when I am doing twice as much as anybody
else. Anybody who looks carefully could see me
shouting that belief that underlies my illness
style").

Health Style

Flip to the health side of your paper. Find a clean space
to start thinking about your wellness style.

1) Recall three stimulating times for you and make a note
of them.

Note: *Again, this is the key question (this and ques-*
tion #3). If people don't get some data down
here, they won't be able to answer the style
questions which follow. Give them time, help
them massage the issue so they can get into it,
but don't accept arguments from the audience.

2) Mark down some words that describe what stimulating
is for you. As you look at your three examples, what
is "stimulating" like for you?

3) Recall a significant healing experience in which you
were involved.

Note: *Give people some time for this, then answer the*
puzzled looks by saying something like, "Any
healing experience. Most healing experiences
(if not all) go both ways. It doesn't matter
which kind of experience you pick. Take one
that crosses your mind first."

4) Surround that experience with the process and feelings
that were active. What were the dynamics? What kind
of healing mechanisms were involved? People? Machi-
nery? Where did the healing take place? How did it
take place? It was healing from what to what?

We can't ask all the questions, but make some notes
on the dynamics of that healing experience for you.

5) Based on what you're in touch with as you consider
your healing experience, make a comment on your style

of healing by saying, "Based on this example, my style
of healing is _____."

6) Draw a picture of yourself being really well.

   *Note: People will generally laugh a little. Encourage
   them to get into it by just starting their
   scribbles at random and seeing what they come
   up with. Give them plenty of time so that they
   can include details in the picture (other people,
   faces, and so forth), but don't tell them what
   to put into their pictures.*

7) Take a look at your picture and write down one summary
   word for the essence of the wellness that you see in
   that picture. Write down a summary word that catches
   the feeling tone of wellness for you.

8) When did you feel most like that word today? When did
   you feel most well today? When did you feel most like
   that word?

   *Note: The point here is to connect the image of that
   word with the image of wellness. Make sure
   that you help people make that connection.*

9) List two favors that you could do for yourself yet
   today that would help you feel more like that word,
   that would help you feel more well.

   *Note: Again, you're trying to help people make the
   bridge between their summary word and what wellness means to them. Encourage people to list
   small favors they could do for themselves, not
   major projects.*

General Insights From These Questions

Compare and contrast your sickness style and your wellness
style.

*Note: These three closing questions are the important ele-
ment. Here people are trying to milk the insights
about themselves from what they have just done.
Give them plenty of time, perhaps even some examples.*

1) Take a look at your two pictures (your picture of you
   being sick and your picture of you being well) and make
   some observations to yourself about what you see when
   you compare them.

2) Look at your two words (your summary word for sickness and your summary word for wellness). Make some observations about how those words do, or do not, fit together. Make some observations about how those two words are related.

3) Take a minute or two to look over all of your answers and write down any insights which strike you about you, your style, and the ways you contribute both to your sickness and to your wellness.

> *Note:* *Give people a fair amount of time to do this, so that they milk all the observations they can from it. Perhaps, ask them to number the observations and come up with three to five specific ideas that strike them.*
>
> *When participants have had ample time for this question, proceed with Step #3 (page 38) of the process and divide participants into small groups for discussion. See the exercise process notes.*

SELF-CARE

11. THE MARATHON STRATEGY (p 49)

   This chalk talk utilizes the metaphor of a marathon to
   demonstrate that over the "long run" those who care for
   themselves and take time to stop and fill up along the
   way finish the race with gusto to spare. (15 minutes)

12. DAILY RITUALS (p 54)

   This short exercise helps participants identify and rate
   their small daily rituals that accompany wake-up time,
   lunch-time, dinner/evening-time and bed-time.
   (10-15 minutes)

13. LETTER FROM THE INTERIOR (p 56)

   Participants explore the impact of physical self-care
   practices by writing a letter from their body detailing
   all of its complaints and commendations. (20-30 minutes)

14. THE LAST MEAL (p 58)

   Participants record and analyze the quality and quantity
   consumed at their last meal. (15-30 minutes)

15. THE EXERCISE EXERCISE (p 62)

   This short group exercise routine, complete from warm-up
   to cool down, will get the group "psyched" for learning.
   (15 minutes)

16. SANCTUARY (p 67)

   This technique demonstrates the use of an imagery "sanctuary" or brief retreat from daily stresses. (15-30 minutes)

17. MARCO POLO (p 70)

   This thought-provoking short film and self-analysis process
   allows participants to explore the issue of mental health
   from the viewpoint of a young child. (15-20 minutes)

18. DISCRIMINATING FEELER (p 74)

   This exercise explores the importance of feelings in mental
   health, emotions that might be aroused in specific situations and personal feeling preferences and patterns.
   (30-45 minutes)

19. INTERPERSONAL NEEDS/SATISFACTIONS (p 81)

   In this exercise participants examine their social networks and analyze how well their interpersonal needs are
   being met. (60-90 minutes)

20. IRISH SWEEPSTAKES (p 90)

    Participants plan a budget for their million dollar sweep-
    stakes win and examine the implied values.   (20-30 minutes)

21. SPIRITUAL PILGRIMAGE (p 94)

    This lifeline drawing allows participants an opportunity
    to trace their spiritual journey, and discover how it
    contributes to their well-being.   (20-30 minutes)

11 THE MARATHON STRATEGY

This chalk talk utilizes the metaphor of a marathon to demonstrate that over the "long run" those who care for themselves and take time to stop and fill up along the way finish the race with gusto to spare. Participants are asked to identify the personal nourishment they need for sustenance along life's way.

GOALS

1) To help participants recognize that they cannot make it all the way through life without nourishing themselves.

2) To help participants identify the personal energizers they can utilize to refill themselves.

GROUP SIZE

Any size group is appropriate. This chalk talk is particularly effective with large audiences.

TIME FRAME

15 minutes

MATERIALS NEEDED

A "Marathon Strategy" worksheet for each participant; blackboard or newsprint easel.

PROCESS

1) The trainer introduces the marathon metaphor, using the blackboard to illustrate and diagram some or all of the following points:

 • Marathon distances vary with each sport:

running	26 miles
cross country skiing	35 miles
bicycling	150-200 miles
swimming	8-10 miles

The distance for each sport is calculated at about 25% further than a person can normally go with the energy that was stored in his body at the start of the race. This is what makes a marathon so difficult. Unless the racer takes on nourishment along the way, he "runs out of gas" before the end!

● When the readily available store of carbohydrates/glycogen are burned up, the body must make a painful and dramatic shift and begin to convert protein from the muscle tissue to burn for energy. Marathon competitors label this experience "hitting the wall." Hitting the wall doesn't simply mean you're more tired than before. It means the body has depleted its readily available energy resources and must begin "stealing" energy from the muscles themselves. This depleted condition usually is signaled by pain, and a loss of orientation -- sometimes complete collapse.

		The wall	
running	0	18 miles	26 miles
X-C skiing	0	25 miles	35 miles
bicycling	0	125 miles	150-200 miles
swimming	0	6 miles	8-10 miles

● Since you cannot make it all the way to the finish line without completely depleting your store of glycogen, "food stations" are set up along the way to allow competitors to replenish. By taking in carbohydrates in a variety of forms along the way, well-conditioned competitors can reach the finish without "hitting the wall."

● Since it takes 20 to 30 minutes for the body to process nutrients, the most important food station is the first. The next most important, the second, and so on. By the time you reach the last food station the nourishment you swallow won't take effect until after you finish. If you do hit the wall, you probably won't die! At worst, you'll roll belly up in the grass and get carried away on a stretcher. At best, you'll have to stop and walk for 20 minutes while 500 or 1,000 people pass you by, until the new nourishment enters your system.

Even experienced marathoners need to memorize these facts and remind themselves each race to stop and replenish from the very beginning, because at the first and the second feed stations a conditioned athlete won't "feel" the need for nourishment.

The racer's perceived level of energy over the

course of a marathon follows a pattern similar to
the one below.

*Note: The trainer will want to draw this graph
         on the board.*

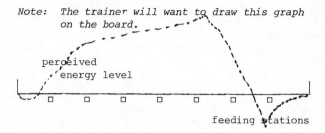

At the beginning, having rested a few days before,
the racer's energy may be low. But it rises,
until at the mid-point of a race most well-conditioned competitors feel a rush of energy. They
feel as if they could go forever! Beware! When
the energy feels the highest, that is the very
time when new nourishment must be taken in
to avoid a collapse later.

• The marathon metaphor applies to more than races
  and to more than physical stamina. We can't get
  through life maintaining a high level of vitality
  without receiving energy-replenishing nourishment
  along the way. We, too, must memorize the fact
  that when we are "flying high" with energy, we
  must stop to care for ourselves, and replenish
  our energy in all dimensions of life. Rather than
  ignore our personal needs when we feel good, we
  want to memorize the fact that our "high" is a
  sure signal that we need to stop and fill up.
  Those who don't, hit the wall and burn out.

  *Note: The trainer will want to give examples of
          this phenomenon such as the need for nur-
          turing relationships while they're still
          vibrant.*

• At most marathon feeding stations participants
  are offered a standard fare of water, gatorade,
  erg, orange slices and granola bars. But in real
  life physical nourishment is only one of our
  sources of energy replenishment. To go the distance we need to tune in to our own needs in all
  areas so that we know what will be satisfying
  fillers for us.

2) The trainer distributes a "Marathon Strategy" work-

sheet to all participants and helps them to reflect on their own self-care patterns and needs, asking them to identify their own personal "fillers" and "energizers" -- the nourishers that sustain them over the "long-run" of life.

Note: *The trainer can help people focus on their fillers by asking questions such as:*

> * *What life experiences fill your heart?*
> * *What nourishes your self-concept? Your capacity to love?*
> * *What nurtures your creativity? Your productivity?*
> * *What people/places/activities energize you?*
> * *When you feel depleted what restores you?*

> *The trainer may also want to give several examples of energizers such as watching a sun rise, loving hugs, compliments from my boss, a long leisurely walk, taking a course, playing the piano, etc.*

Participants stock their feeding stations by writing down several personal energizers and fillers at each food stop.

3) The trainer asks for examples of personal "nourishers" at each "feeding station" and records these on the board. This allows participants to be stimulated by the ideas and insights of others.

TRAINER'S NOTES

MARATHON STRATEGY WORKSHEET

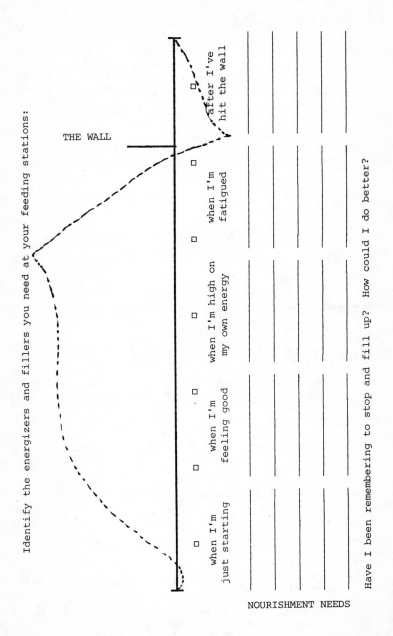

12 DAILY RITUALS

This short exercise helps participants identify and rate their small daily rituals that accompany wake-up time, lunch-time, dinner/evening time and bed-time. Participants identify at least one uplifter for each period of the day.

GOALS

1) To highlight personal awareness of daily patterns.

2) To identify a sure-fire energizer for each period of the day.

GROUP SIZE

Any size group is appropriate.

TIME FRAME

10-15 minutes

MATERIALS NEEDED

Blank paper for each participant.

PROCESS

1) The trainer points out that our days are filled with personal rituals such as brushing teeth, combing hair, reading the newspaper, a noon walk, stretching, smoking, drinking coffee, driving the same route at the same time every day, watching the evening news, loading the dishwasher, asking the kids about school, etc. Most of these we repeat day after day.

The trainer asks participants to reflect on their personal rituals -- patterned behaviors they repeat almost every day and to list four or five for each of these time periods:

☐ early morning rituals
☐ noon-time rituals
☐ evening/dinner-time rituals
☐ bed-time rituals

2) The trainer points out that some of these rituals are positive uplifters, some are negative drainers and others may appear neutral. Participants are asked to

quickly rate each of the 15-20 rituals they've listed according to the following scale:

+2 -- a high vitality energizer
+1 -- generally an uplifter
 0 -- neutral/practical necessity
-1 -- slight drainer
-2 -- definitely a downer

3) Participants then select one sure-fire, quick-fix energizer for each period of the day. They may select from their list or write down anything new that occurs to them.

4) The trainer asks the participants to share their very best high vitality rituals for each period of the day with the whole group. The trainer records the suggestions on the blackboard and encourages participants to listen to the suggestions of others and make notes of any they particularly want to remember.

5) The trainer challenges the group to be sure to engage in each of their sure-fire energizers every day without exception, and to notice, as well as appreciate the small spark of energy each provides.

VARIATION

- As part of Step #5, the trainer may instruct each person in the group to take the next 2 minutes and engage in their personal "quick-fix" appropriate to that time of day, then return.

Be sure to attend to the dynamics that occur and when all have returned comment on what you observed.

TRAINER'S NOTES

13 LETTER FROM THE INTERIOR

Participants explore the impact of physical self-care
practices by writing a letter from their body detailing
all of its complaints and commendations.

GOALS

1) To heighten awareness of physical self-care patterns
    and their impact on well-being.

2) To target specific negative self-care habits that need
    modification.

3) To reinforce positive self-care practices.

GROUP SIZE

Unlimited; easily adapted for use with individuals

TIME FRAME

20-30 minutes

MATERIALS NEEDED

A blank sheet of paper for each participant

*Note: This exercise is most effective when preceded by some
form of self-care assessment and/or body awareness
experience.*

PROCESS

1) The trainer asks participants to reflect on how well
    they've been treating their bodies lately, asking
    questions such as:

    □ How well have you been taking care of your body
      in the past few months, weeks, days, hours?

    □ What have you been <u>putting into</u> your body (eating,
      drinking, smoking, medication, etc) that may
      diminish or enhance your health?

    □ What have you been <u>doing to</u> your body (pace, work-
      load, pressure, stimulation, medical self-care, etc)
      that promotes or inhibits well-being?

□ What have you been <u>doing with</u> your body (exercise, sloth, play, strain, etc) that result in positive or negative consequences?

□ How well have you been letting your body rest?

2) Once the group is warmed up to the issue of physical self-care, the trainer distributes blank sheets of paper to all participants and asks them to write a letter from their body about the care it's been receiving. The trainer gives instructions something like this:

● Write a letter from your body to yourself. Take a whole page or two. Let your body say all it wants you to hear.

● Start by writing: "Dear (your name)."
Then start reporting your body's positive and negative reactions to your self-care patterns. What does your body want to say about how you exercise it, what you feed it, rest time, play time? What special favors does your body really appreciate? Is one part of your body experiencing pain? Give it a voice!

   Note: The trainer may want to give some humorous and serious examples such as "Dear Sue, Ouch! What are you doing to me? Why do I have to carry all your problems around for you? Please let me put them down once in a while! Your Aching Back." Or, "Dear Joe, Ten pounds gone -- super! Keep up the good work. Thanks for getting my legs moving again, too!"

● Take plenty of time to tune in to all of the messages your body is trying to send you and start writing. (Allow at least 5 minutes for writing letters.)

3) Each participant finds two others to join her in a trio for sharing. The three people read their letters out loud and discuss them together as a group. (10 minutes)

4) The trainer reconvenes the group and asks for insights and observations.

14 THE LAST MEAL

Participants record and analyze the quality and quantity consumed at their last meal. This exercise is an excellent lead-in for an in-depth presentation on nutrition and health.

GOALS

1) To highlight participants' eating patterns and their effects.

2) To provoke a discussion of positive nutrition habits.

GROUP SIZE

Any size group is appropriate.

TIME FRAME

15 minutes without discussion groups; 30 minutes with discussion groups.

MATERIALS NEEDED

"The Last Meal" worksheets for all participants.

PROCESS

Note: This exercise is particularly effective immediately following a meal-time when participants may have lost control and "pigged out" or eaten too little to satisfy their hunger.

1) The trainer distributes "The Last Meal" worksheets to all participants and asks them to write down in the left column everything they ate and drank at the last meal (including any pre or post-meal snacks!).

Participants estimate the nutritional value of each item in the second column and record the appropriate calorie count in the third column.

Note: The trainer may want to stop here and provide specific information on the nutritional and caloric content of foods, but it is not essential. It may even be advantageous for people to become aware of their nutritional information deficit.

2) The next three columns on the worksheet focus on the process rather than the content of the meal. The trainer asks people to think back to the meal and picture it as vividly as possible in their imagination, then try to remember how each different food tasted, noting it in column #4.

The trainer next directs participants' attention to their eating style. Was it hurried? Distracted? Emotional? People jot down comments on their eating style.

3) The trainer asks participants to answer the questions at the bottom of the worksheet and summarize their insights about the last meal.

4) The trainer will want to supplement this process exercise with accurate information on healthy diet, calorie intake, nutritional balance, as well as a discussion of healthy eating styles. Participants can then compare their own behaviors (as recorded on the worksheet) against the "Healthy Standards" as presented by the trainer.

5) The trainer may ask for comments and observations from the group, or divide participants into buzz groups (4-6 persons) for discussion of their personal insights and observations about their nutrition habits.

TRAINER'S NOTES

Adapted from the Wellaware program developed at Miller-Dwan Hospital, Duluth MN.

THE LAST MEAL

Type and Amount of Food Eaten	Estimated Nutritional Analysis	Approx Calorie Count	Comments on Taste

How did this meal differ from my usual meal?

My nutrition grade for this meal _____.

If I kept this eating pattern up for the next 5 years what would I look like?   What would I feel like?

What I'd like to change:

Comments on Eating Style	How does my body feel about what I ate and how I ate it?

Comments and reactions:

What does eating mean to me?

15 THE EXERCISE EXERCISE

This short group exercise routine, complete from warm-up to cool down, will get the group "psyched" for learning. It will energize them!

GOALS

1) To demonstrate the benefits of exercise -- fun, exhiliration and stress reduction.

2) To rejuvenate participants.

3) To teach target pulse monitoring of aerobic exercise.

GROUP SIZE

The more people, the merrier, as long as each person has a 4' X 4' area of floor space.

TIME FRAME

Approximately 15 minutes.

MATERIALS NEEDED

Cassette player and tape with movement music.

PROCESS

1) The trainer introduces the session by having participants get comfortable for movement . . . loosen belts; unbutton shirt collars; take off suit coats; take off heeled shoes; etc. Invite people to stand and prepare for fitness fun.

It's helpful if the trainer briefly explains what the group will be doing -- a stretch out, a moderate aerobic routine and a cool-down routine. Mention the goals of the session in a light-mannered way.

2) As the trainer leads the group through the stretch-out routine (Step #3) she describes the benefits of aerobic exercise and teaches the target pulse measurement method as outlined below.

- The pain, torture and agony many of us experienced in the old school of physical education was probably due to not taking the time to properly warm-up our bodies before engaging in vigorous exercise and from working out too hard.

- The warm-up and cool-down segments of exercise are just as important as the aerobic portion.

- To reap all the physical benefits of exercise, three important factors must be adhered to:

Duration - you need to exercise at least 20 minutes at a time.

Intensity - here's where that wonderful word aerobic comes in. Aerobic simply means "with oxygen." Aerobic exercise includes any activities that force your body to process large amounts of oxygen. Our muscles need oxygen to function and this oxygen demand goes up dramatically when we work them. As you exercise harder, you need more oxygen and the heart rate goes up. By monitoring your heart rate (pulse-monitored exercise) you can indirectly measure how hard you're working out.

Note: *You will need to stop the warm-up stretches for a few moments to explain and demonstrate pulse-monitored exercise.*

   First instruct participants in taking their pulse (at wrist or side of neck, with first two fingers, not thumb; count for 10 seconds and multiply by six; the first beat is counted as zero). Have everyone take their resting pulse and write it down.

   Next tell participants how to figure their maximum heart rate (220 minus their age) and write it down.

   For regular, aerobic exercise, basically healthy people should work out at 70% to 85% of their maximum heart rate.

   People with health problems may need to work out at a lower rate. Check with your physician if you have any questions about the level of exercise appropriate for you.

   For this demonstration, participants will calculate their target pulse as 80% of maximum. Ask them to calculate their aerobic target pulse (maximum heart rate figured above multiplied by .8). For example, a 26 year old would have a maximum heart rate of 194 beats per minute (220 minus 26). He should exercise aerobically at about 156 (194 X .8) beats per minute.

It's best to check pulse at least twice during an exercise routine to determine when aerobic levels are reached.

Frequency - fitness experts recommend aerobic exercise at least three times per week; four times per week is better; five or six times per week is great!

● One of the most important aspects of exercise is consistency -- keeping exercise in your schedule. In order for this to happen, exercise needs to be enjoyable.

The popularity of aerobic dance programs bears witness to the importance of having fun. Aerobic dance is one way to make healthful self-care fun! Exercising to music with a group of people adds a new element of excitement to the workout.

3) As the trainer describes the benefits of aerobic exercise, participants can join in these warm-up movements that comprise the stretch-out section of the routine.

Warm-ups can be done in any order. All movements should be performed at a slow relaxed pace; stretch gently, don't strain; stretching should feel good, not painful; hold the stretch; don't bounce.

Note: Some people may have difficulty with a few of these stretches. Encourage everyone to approximate the stretch but to go only as far as comfortable for them.

● Head arcs - feet a little more than hip distance apart; keep the stomach tucked in and the butt squeezed tightly; roll head from right shoulder to left shoulder with chin dropped down to your chest; your chin will make a half moon; roll head back from left shoulder to right shoulder. Repeat 4-5 times.

● Shoulder shrugs - feet in same position as above; arms down at sides; raise shoulders up to ears and release. Repeat 4-5 times.

- Reach and stretch - feet in same position as above; arms down at sides; raise shoulders up to ears and release. Repeat 4-5 times.

- Side stretches - feet in same position as above; with right arm overhead and left arm down at left side, reach right arm to the left as you lean from the waist to the left side; repeat with left arm overhead and right arm down to the side as you lean to the right. Repeat 4-5 times.

- Floor touchers - with feet about four inches apart and toes straight ahead, bend over in slow, relaxed manner, rolling down each vertebra as you reach for the floor with your hands; hold for two counts and slowly roll up each vertebra until standing upright again. Repeat 4-5 times.

- Hamstring stretch - with feet slightly further apart than hips and arms out to side at shoulder height, bend forward with straight flat back and straight legs; keep head up; look forward; hold; come back to starting position. Repeat 3-5 times.

- Knee hugs - with feet slightly apart, lift your right knee to your chest; use your hands to pull it up and in; be gentle. Hold for 10-15 seconds.

- Ankle circles - with feet slightly apart and left hand on hip, lift right leg as if to climb a steep stair, grasping the shin just below the knee with your right hand; circle the right ankle clockwise 5-7 times, counter clockwise 5-7 times. Repeat with left leg and ankle.

4) The trainer teaches the group a simple aerobic dance routine she has choreographed beforehand to fit the music.

   Note: The most effective way to teach a dance routine is to start with one pattern, do it with the music, add another pattern, do both with the music and so on until the whole routine is completed.

   Don't try to teach a complicated dance sequence in a limited time frame. Three or four steps is plenty. Or make up a routine that uses jogging in place, polka steps, jumping jacks and other familiar movements.

Participants should take a pulse check before the routine and immediately on completion.

5) After 5-6 minutes of vigorous exercise, the trainer leads participants through a cool-down and stretch-out period using the movements outlined in Step #3.

Everyone should check her pulse periodically until it returns to the original resting level. The trainer may ask participants to record the highest pulse rate they experienced during the exercise routine and the time elapsed after exercise until the pulse returned to its resting rate.

VARIATIONS

■ In Step #4 small groups of participants can work together and make up their own routine. The trainer provides music and ideas for movement, if needed.

Music is key to the success of aerobic dance. Soundtracks from popular films, swing or jazz and light rock are especially energizing. Experiment with different tempos and moods. Check your local library for free records and tapes of all kinds of music. The YMCA Fitness Fantasia program (PO Box 25099, Colorado Spring CO 80936) suggests these selections:

warm-up and stretch out:
* "Reach Out and Touch" (Diana Ross)
* "Everyday Man" (BJ Thomas)
* "Just the Two of Us" (Grover Washington Jr)
moderate aerobic routine:
* "Greatest American Hero" (Mike Post)
stretch-out and cool-down:
* "We've Got Tonight" (Kenny Rogers & Sheenah Easton)
* "The Rose" (Bette Midler)
* "Love Theme from 'An Officer and a Gentleman'" (Lee Ritenour)

TRAINER'S NOTES

Submitted by Linda Nowobielski

16 SANCTUARY

This technique demonstrates the use of an imagery "sanctuary" or brief retreat from daily stresses. This process
may be used as part of a guided fantasy or as a tool for
persons having trouble sleeping.

GOALS

1)   To demonstrate the vivid and powerful effects of
     relaxing imagery.

2)   To give the participants a pleasant self-induced focus
     of attention for relaxation training.

GROUP SIZE

Unlimited; easy to use with individuals as well.

TIME FRAME

Approximately 15-30 minutes.

PROCESS

1)   Participants are instructed to find a comfortable,
     balanced posture (arms and legs uncrossed), reclining
     in a chair or on the floor. Participants are encour-
     aged to close their eyes as the trainer gives a series
     of basic relaxation suggestions (slow, deep breathing;
     centering techniques; calming phrases; etc)

2)   Once participants begin to shift their focus of aware-
     ness inside, the trainer asks them to visualize in
     their mind's eye a large movie screen, noting the top,
     bottom, sides and texture of the screen.

3)   The trainer briefly describes a "sanctuary" as a
     special personal place to which an individual can
     travel for a brief respite; a place where you can
     relax, enjoy your leisure and learn in your own way
     how to take time out from the stimulation that crowds
     your life.

4)   The trainer then asks participants to focus on their
     movie screen and wait for such a personal sanctuary
     to appear. The place that begins to take shape on
     the screen in each participant's mind may be a real
     or mythical setting. It may be out in nature or

inside a healing temple from ages ago.

The trainer suggests that participants <u>allow</u> the image to form and not try to force it in any way.

5) As the scene becomes clearer for participants, the trainer suggests that they "step into" the scene. Once inside the scene they may attend with great curiosity and detail to the sensory qualities of the place: gentle sounds, peaceful silence, fragrances, breezes, textures, colors, shapes.

Participants are to explore their sanctuary space with all of their senses until it becomes vivid and complete, enjoying the calm and quiet.

6) When the time allotted to this exercise is almost over the trainer suggests that since participants now know the way to this special place, they may return at any time they wish. Participants are then asked to temporarily say goodbye to their sanctuary and return to the room.

   Note: The trainer may suggest that when using this technique in the future participants may want to set an alarm to call them back from the sanctuary. This will eliminate the need to keep time.

7) The trainer asks for observations and comments from the group. If no one raises the issue, the trainer should ask about sensory phenomena that accompanied the experience such as tingling of the extremeties, lifting sensations, time distortion, etc. Point out that these sensations are evidence of how deeply participants allowed themselves to relax.

VARIATIONS

- The trainer may want to provide some restful musical background to accompany this exercise. Pachelbel's Canon in D or nature sounds work well.

- Once participants have envisioned and entered their sanctuary, the trainer may lead them through a structured fantasy that further focuses their attention on this special place. Or the trainer may suggest that participants meet their own "guide" who will take them on a tour of their sanctuary.

■ A group of five or six participants could form a pinwheel
  arrangement, lying or reclining with all heads in the
  center. From this position they can mutually create and
  share aloud a sanctuary for their group.

TRAINER'S NOTES

Submitted by David X Swenson

17 MARCO POLO

This thought-provoking short film and self-analysis process allows participants to explore the issue of mental health from the viewpoint of a young child.

GOALS

1) To rediscover childlike qualities of mental health.

2) To identify strategies for recapturing/increasing desired characteristics.

GROUP SIZE

Unlimited

TIME FRAME

15-20 minutes

MATERIALS NEEDED

The film, "YOU"   (Available from The Cally Curtis Co, 1111 N Las Palmas Ave, Hollywood CA 90038, 213/467-1101; $75/rental, $225/purchase)
"Self-Analysis" worksheet for each participant.

PROCESS

1) The trainer introduces the film, "YOU," indicating that a lively mind is an essential component of well-being from a whole person perspective.

2) The film is viewed by all.

Note: This four minute film shows a seven month old baby exploring the living room and highlights the value of curiosity, enthusiasm, energy and openness to new experiences. The film ends with the question, "Are there any characteristics of your younger days you'd like to recapture?"

3) The trainer reviews the film content and elicits discussion of the major points.

Note: The Meeting Guide which accompanies the film offers excellent suggestions for stimulating group discussion.

4) The trainer distributes the "Self-Analysis" worksheets and asks participants to reflect on their own "mental" health as portrayed in the film. The trainer may want to walk through the worksheet, giving examples along the way and especially encouraging people to think of at least 5-10 ideas for recapturing/increasing each desirable quality.

5) The trainer asks for insights from the total group concerning strategies for enhancing mental health.

6) Participants may share with the group one or two of their resolutions concerning what they will do today to exercise their childlike qualities.

VARIATION

After Step #4, participants could form small groups for discussion of self-analysis profiles. After each person has shared, the small group could brainstorm strategies for recapturing/increasing the identified qualities. Allow 10-15 additional minutes for this variation.

TRAINER'S NOTES

SELF-ANALYSIS WORKSHEET

1)   In watching the film "YOU," what three qualities of your
      personality as a child did you recognize as your "best?"

      _____

      _____

      _____

2)   Which of these do you consider most valuable today? Put
      the three qualities in priority order then answer the
      questions for each characteristic:

My most valuable childlike quality

#1 _____

      a)   Am I as (quality #1) as I once was?   ☐ yes   ☐ no

      b)   If not, why not? If so, how come?

      c)   How would my life be better today if I were more
           (quality #1)?

      d)   How could I recapture/increase my (quality #1)?

      e)   What will I do today?

My second most valuable childlike quality

#2 _____

    a) Am I as (quality #2) as I once was? ☐ yes ☐ no

    b) If not, why not? If so, how come?

    c) How would my life be better today if I were more
       (quality #2)?

    d) How could I recapture/increase my (quality #2)?

    e) What will I do today?

My third most valuable childlike quality

#3 _____

    a) Am I as (quality #3) as I once was? ☐ yes ☐ no

    b) If not, why not? If so, how come?

    c) How would my life be better today if I were more
       (quality #3)?

    d) How could I recapture/increase my (quality #3)?

    e) What will I do today?

18 THE DISCRIMINATING FEELER

This three part exercise includes an introductory chalk talk on the importance of feelings in mental health, a large group brainstorming of emotions that might be aroused in specific situations and small group exploration of personal feeling preferences and patterns.

GOALS

1) To help participants expand their vocabulary of feeling words.

2) To explore emotional responses to a variety of situations.

3) To identify personal response styles and consider other options.

GROUP SIZE

Unlimited

TIME FRAME

30-45 minutes

MATERIALS NEEDED

Blackboard or newsprint easel
"Feeling Vignettes" and "Feeling Words" list

PROCESS

1) The trainer introduces mental health as an essential area for exploration in wellness promotion and explains the importance of feelings as a component of mental health. The trainer may want to incorporate the following points in this introduction:

    a) Mentally healthy people are characterized by . . .
        * capacity to feel deeply
        * sensitivity to feelings in themselves and others
        * willingness to experience feelings
        * appropriate expression of a wide range of feelings

    b) As human beings we are created with a capacity to feel a wide spectrum of emotions from irritation to

rage, delight to exhiliration. Yet most people
limit themselves to a narrow range because . . .
* we want to limit "bad" feelings and only
  experience "good" emotions (or vice versa) and
  consequently spend a good deal of energy "keeping the lid on" feelings rather than exploring
  the limits of our emotional capacity;
* we confuse experiencing an emotion with expressing it or acting on it and thus we shut off
  our anger (or sexual attraction) before we
  feel it fully because we fear the implications
  of expressing those feelings;
* most of us lack the vocabulary to distinguish
  and describe the subtle shades of our emotional
  experience.

2) The trainer reads one of the "Feelings Vignettes"
   (p 77) asking participants to tune into themselves
   and imagine how they might feel in that situation.

3) The trainer solicits from the group eight to ten
   examples of different (or similar) feeling responses
   to the situation and writes these feeling words on the
   blackboard commenting on the variety of reactions and
   differences between people's experiences.

   *Note: The trainer may want to group the responses
   in categories that illustrate shades of meaning in a general feeling tone.*

4) The trainer reads several more vignettes, following
   the process outlined in Steps #2 and #3, again highlighting the diversity of response.

   *Note: Some groups may need help zeroing in on nuances
   of feeling. If three people in a row respond
   with "upset," (or a similar vague feeling), the
   trainer can nudge participants by asking for
   clarification -- "Do you mean anxious? or
   worried? or irritated?" etc). If a group
   really gets stuck, the trainer can ask them to
   imagine all the different emotions people might
   have in response to the situation. (How would
   your mother react? A favorite teacher? A
   child? etc.)*

5) When a substantial collection of feeling words has
   been collected on the board, the trainer can ask the
   group to add even more feeling words to fill in the
   holes, brainstorming together until the list includes
   80 words or more.

> *Note: See the "Feeling Words" list (pp 78-79) for*
> *ideas if the group gets stuck.*

6) Participants are asked to jot down their own five
    favorite and five least favorite feelings.

7) Participants divide into groups of four (or rejoin
    previous groups). The trainer asks each group to come
    to a consensus on their top five favorite emotions and
    their five least favorite feelings. (10 minutes)

> *Note: The trainer may want to remind group members*
> *of the good listening rules and encourage*
> *groups to make sure that all opinions receive*
> *serious consideration in the consensus process.*

VARIATIONS

At the end of this exercise the trainer may wish to challenge participants to undertake a three-step feelings
awareness experiment:

- choose one or two feelings you would like to be more
  open to;
- commit yourself to search out at least two opportunities to experience that emotion;
- notice the outcome when you allow yourself to experience
  the feeling fully.

If this is an ongoing wellness course participants could
report on the experiment at the next group meeting.

TRAINER'S NOTES

FEELING VIGNETTES

You wake up in the night and hear a strange noise . . .

You are rocking gently with a young child on your lap . . .

You are watching the state basketball championship. The game
    is tied with three seconds to go and your team has the
    ball . . .

You discover your child has just shoplifted something . . .

You are talking with an employee about her performance, know-
    ing that you have to fire her . . .

You get a letter from your father . . .

The car in front of you is going 50 mph in a 55 mile zone.
    There's no place to pass . . .

You overhear a friend gossiping with a third person about
    you . . .

You step on the scale . . .

Someone you love touches you . . .

You are sitting in the lounge waiting for word from surgery . . .

You watch your child perform in a talent show . . .

The Sears Credit Department calls for the third time this
    week asking for payment on your bill . . .

A person you find attractive sits down next to you at a
    party . . .

You walk through the door on the first day of your new job . . .

You walk through the door on the last day of your job . . .

A friend tells you what a wonderful person you are . . .

Your spouse is angry with you and so upset and frustrated
    when you answer back that he strides out, slamming the
    door so hard the house shakes . . .

Your teenager comes home from school and says "hello" with
    warmth and enthusiasm . . .

You have just spilled your drink on the carpet . . .

FEELING WORDS LIST

acceptance	comfortable	exasperated
admiring	confusion	excited
adored	consoled	exhausted
affectionate	contemptuous	expectant
aggravated	cornered	
alarmed	courageous	faith in
alert	coveting	fearful
alienated	crushed	fed up
amazed	curious	fond
ambivalent	cynical	forlorn
amused		frantic
angry	daring	friendly
annoyed	defeated	frightened
antagonistic	degraded	frustration
anticipating	dejected	fulfilled
anxious	delighted	furious
apathetic	dependent	futility
appalled	depressed	
appealing	despair	glad
appreciated	desperate	gleeful
apprehensive	despised	gloomy
ashamed	devastated	good
assured	disappointed	grateful
astonished	disapproval	great
audacious	disconcerted	grieved
awed	disconsolate	grouchy
	discouraged	grumpy
bashful	disgruntled	guilty
belligerent	disgusted	
benevolent	dislike	happy
bewildered	dismal	hate
bitter	dismayed	helpless
bold	dissatisfied	hopeful
bored	distrustful	hopeless
bothered	disturbed	horrified
bouyant	doubtful	hostile
brave	dour	humbled
bright	down	humiliated
burned up	dread	hurt
calm	eager	
cared-for	edgy	
cautious	elated	
cocky	embarrassed	
competent	enraged	
concern about	envious	
concern for	esteemed	
confident	estranged	

impatient
important
idolized
inadequate
independent
indifferent
indignant
ineffectual
infatuated
inferior
inhibited
inquisitive
irritated
insecure
insulted

jealous
jittery
jolly
jumpy

lethargic
listless
loathed
lonely
longing
lost
love
loved
loyal
lust

mad
meaningless
melancholy
miserable
mistrustful
mixed up
moody

nervous
nosey

optimistic
out of place
outraged
overwhelmed

pained
panicky
passionate

patient
peaceful
perplexed
pessimistic
pitiful
pleased
pressured
proud
provoked
put down
puzzled

refreshed
regretful
rejected
relaxed
relieved
reluctant
repulsed
resentful
resigned
restless
risking

sad
satisfaction
scared
self-conscious
sexy
shocked
shy
skeptical
solemn
sorry
startled
strong
stubborn
sullen
supported
surprised
suspicious
sympathetic

teed-off
tender
tense
tempted
threatened
thrilled
timid
torn up

tough
tranquil
trapped
trepidation
troubled
trusting
turned off
turned on

uncomfortable
uneasy
unfulfilled
unhappy
unsure
untroubled
unwanted
upset
uptight
used
useless

valiant
valued
vibrant
vital
vulnerable

warmth
weak
weary
wonder
worn out
worried
worthless
worthy
wounded
wrung out

yearning

zealous

19 INTERPERSONAL NEEDS/SATISFACTIONS

In this exercise participants generate an overall list of people with whom they relate. They then examine their social connections in light of the demands and rewards inherent in various levels of relationships. Utilizing the "Interpersonal Needs/Satisfactions Grid" participants examine the quality of their current relationship in light of how satisfactorily each relationship meets their need for support and nurture. Following small group discussion of issues and insights raised by the worksheet, each participant identifies two or three persons they wish to recruit into their support network.

GOALS

1) To highlight the variety of intensity and purpose that exists within relationships.

2) To assist individuals in recognizing their interpersonal needs, and to identify the various sources of their support.

3) To motivate participants to be intentional in building a support network that nurtures them at many levels of need.

GROUP SIZE

Unlimited; this exercise is appropriate for both small group settings and large gatherings of 200 or more, as long as the space and timing permit the formation of four person sharing groups.

TIME FRAME

60-90 minutes

MATERIALS NEEDED

A copy of the "Interpersonal Needs/Satisfactions Grid" for each participant.

PROCESS

1) The trainer may wish to open the exercise by discussing the importance of supportive interpersonal relationships and their health enhancing potential. Concepts may include:

- Everyone needs to be appreciated, know fully, loved and valued. Everyone needs to belong.

- Most people are not very intentional in seeking and forming fulfilling relationships and in building their support network. They relate by chance, more often than by choice.

- To be supported, people must be willing to risk opening themselves and stating clearly what they need and want. Guessing games never work out very well for either the giver or the receiver.

A.   THE WIDE NETWORK OF RELATIONSHIPS (15-20 minutes)

2) The trainer asks participants to make a list of people they relate to -- as many as possible in 3-5 minutes. The trainer encourages them to think of many groups -- close family, distant relatives, old school friends, work associates, club or church members, service personnel, etc. -- and to list the names of specific people as quickly as possible.

3) Following the exercise the trainer asks participants for observations . . . and reactions.

4) The trainer may announce that this is a contest -- the winner being the one who listed the most names.

Take a vote --

□ How many listed more than 20? 50? 100? etc.

□ Notice who listed more names on the average. Men? or Women? What's the significance?

□ Determine a male winner and a female winner.

□ Ask them to come forward and each to describe the types of groups they noted.

□ Write out a certificate for the winners or read a commendation similar to these examples:

"We hereby honor (woman) as honorary state senator. Rumor has it she has kissed more babies, shaken more hands, held more heads, had more tears shed on her shoulders, knows more people, has given more favors than anyone else here."

*"We hereby honor (man) honorary father figure
(or chairman of the board). He has mentored more
people, remembered more names, changed more
diapers, scheduled more meetings, returned more
phone calls, volunteered more time, coached more
little league baseball than anyone here."*

□ Present a clever award to each winner, utilizing
materials on hand in the room such as:

* an ash tray -- "To hold your ashes after you
        burn out"
* a pitcher of water -- 1/2 full, 1/2 empty
* a candle, burning on both ends
* a pack of sugar -- "Because you're so sweet"
* a cup of coffee -- "Because we know you gave
        yours away"

B. THE REWARDS AND DEMANDS IN RELATIONSHIPS (15-20 minutes)

5) Utilizing the top portion of the "Interpersonal Needs/
Satisfactions Grid" worksheet, the trainer asks participants to list the names of three or four people with
whom they have significant connections (upper left-
hand column labeled "My major social connections").

*Note: Suggest that participants do not select the
most primary relationship in their life, but
that they also do not select insignificant
relationships -- ones of moderate importance
should be the focus here.*

*Vary the length and intensity of this segment
by the number of people listed. If time is
short -- ask participants to complete the exercise with only one person as a focus. They
will still get the point.*

6) The trainer asks participants to focus on the demands
in each relationship.

Ask the following questions one at a time, giving ample
time for participants to reflect and write their
answers in the column labeled "the demands."

□ What demands (requirements) are placed on you in
this relationship? List all you can think of.

□ Who sets this demand as a requirement in the relationship? Answer this question separately for each
demand you identified! Use an "M" for "my requirement," an "O" for the "other's demand" or a "B" for
"both require it."

□ If this requirement were not fulfilled by you what
difference would it make? Would the relationship
still exist? In what form?

□ What observations and insights occur to you in
light of your answers?

7) The trainer asks participants to focus on the rewards
in each relationship. Ask the following questions,
one at a time, giving ample time for participants to
reflect and write their answers in the column labeled
"the rewards."

□ What specific rewards do you expect in each relationship? List as many as you can think of.

□ What percentage of the time does the relationship
give you this reward? (100%? 78%? 10%?)

□ How completely does the reward match up to your
expectations? (100% -- totally rewarding, 50% --
so-so rewarding, 20% -- not usually very rewarding.)

□ Have you ever told the other person directly that
you expect these rewards? Answer for each reward!
Why? Why not?

□ What observations and insights occur to you in
light of your answers?

C. THE SOCIAL NEEDS THAT NURTURE   (15-20 minutes)

8) The trainer points out that relationships fill a
variety of separate personal needs. One at a time
the trainer describes each need listed on the bottom
left side of the "Interpersonal Needs/Satisfactions
Grid" worksheet -- then asks, "Right now in your life
who do you look to primarily to fill this need for
you?" (Participants list one person only.)

□ Listening -- We all need someone to hear us, and
to understand where we're at -- to pay attention
to us. Who in your life right now do you look to

primarily to listen to you?

☐ Emotional Support -- We all not only need someone
to listen to us, we also need someone to accept us,
and tell us we are loved, and that no matter what
happens, we're OK. Who in your life right now do
you primarily look to for emotional support?

☐ Emotional Challenge -- At times, we all need someone to give us feedback, to tell us whether we're
crazy, whether we're misinterpreting -- someone
to hold a mirror up to us and help us see ourselves from the outside. Usually we will allow
people to challenge us and offer us a reality test,
only after they have first listened to us and
accepted us. Who in your life right now do you
primarily look to for this emotional challenge?

☐ Technical Support -- We also need someone to tell
us that we're good at what we do. Whether our pro-
fession is home work or office work, whether we're
paid for our work or not -- we all want someone to
praise us for our skills and for a job well done.
Who in your life right now do you primarily look
to for this technical support?

☐ Technical Stimulation -- In our relationships we
not only need praise, we also need to be challenged
to grow, and stimulated with new ideas. Who in
your life right now do you primarily look to for
this technical stimulation?

☐ Play -- Finally, we all need people to play with.
This is not the competitive play seen in many
athletic contests. The technical word for the
play we have in mind is "to dink around with."
Who in your life right now do you look to primarily
to fool around with -- to play with?

9) The trainer asks participants to complete the "how
successful" column on the worksheet -- by considering
the question, "How successfully does the person you
identified fulfill this need for you?" Use percen-
tages to estimate the answer (10%, 28%, 98%, etc).

10) The trainer asks participants to mark any need that
is not fulfilled at least 75% of the time. For those
needs participants are asked to list two or three
other persons who could potentially help fill this
need. (Be sure participants identify specific people
they know, not broad categories.)

D.   <u>SMALL GROUP SHARING</u>   (20-30 minutes)

11)   The trainer divides participants into groups of four
      persons each (or utilizes previously established dis-
      cussion groups). Participants are instructed to spend
      4-5 minutes each, sharing as much as they like about
      their social needs, and the manner in which these are
      currently being filled. The trainer may encourage par-
      ticipants to look for the following factors:

      ☐ Do you rely on one person primarily for all needs?
        or many different people?

      ☐ Do you ever look for a need to be fulfilled by a
        person unlikely to ever offer you that? Is your
        hope inappropriate? Necessary?

      ☐ What are the similarities and differences among
        members of your group?

      ☐ Who would you like to recruit for your support net-
        work? (two or three people), and how will you plan
        to begin developing this relationship to a greater
        depth after this workshop is over?

E.   <u>PLENARY DISCUSSION</u>   (10 minutes)

12)   Following the sharing in small groups, the trainer
      reconvenes the entire group and asks for observations
      and insights. The following issues may be highlighted
      by the trainer if not expressed by the group. Personal
      examples of each may be elicited as well.

      In re-viewing your support network, keep these prici-
      ples in mind:

      ● It is extremely unlikely that one person can meet
        all of our interpersonal needs. Don't depend on a
        single soul to function as your entire support
        network. If they have a bad day, you get nothing!
        Also, it's a heavy burden to place on someone else.

      ● Frustration results when we expect an inappropriate
        person to meet a particular need. Don't bother
        looking for "listening" from someone you know can't
        or won't come through. Don't wait forever for your
        boss to say, "I love you." Just accept her praise
        of your work and appreciate that!

□ If there's a vacant position (e.g. spouse, best friend, father confessor) in your life for a time that may be disappointing, but you can still find people to meet each of the interpersonal needs.

□ Intentionality is essential in human relationships. Know what you need and then search out someone to help you satisfy that need. You have to reveal yourself to get your needs met. Ask for what you want. It's foolish to say to yourself, "If they really loved me they would know what I want without my asking." It's foolish to make other people guess what you need. When you do, you're less likely to receive what would fill you.

□ It's risky to ask for what you want. Others might not give it to you. Or if they do, you may discover that it's not as satisfying as you had imagined. The risk of rejection and dissatisfaction, however, seem small in comparison to the risk of isolation and frustration.

□ When you find yourself feeling isolated and lonely, it's likely that you're not getting all of what you need from others. It might be necessary for you to acknowledge the support you're missing and to carefully analyze your support network and to recruit people who will fill the gaps in your relationships.

VARIATIONS

■ If time is short, this exercise could be cut to as little as 30 minutes by focusing primarily on Section C "The Social Needs That Nurture."

■ The exercise could be supplemented by a session which helps participants identify and plan steps for the development of a personal support group.

■ The trainer may very well substitute a different list of interpersonal needs, while still utilizing and benefiting from the process as outlined in this exercise.

The "Interpersonal Needs/Satisfactions Grid" is based on research reported by A Pines and E Aronson in Burnout: From Tedium to Personal Growth (New York: The Free Press, 1983).

INTERPERSONAL NEEDS/SATISFACTIONS GRID

MY MAJOR SOCIAL CONNECTIONS

    1)

    2)

    3)

    4)

MY SOCIAL NEEDS   to whom do you look?

    listening

    emotional support

    emotional challenge

    technical support

    technical stimulation

    play

THE DEMANDS   THE REWARDS

how successful?   who else could potentially
                                         fill this need?

20 IRISH SWEEPSTAKES

Participants are told they have won the million dollar
sweepstakes, and are asked to make a plan for the next
year in light of that fact. They write out a budget that
accounts for all the money and then examine the values
imbedded in that budget.

GOALS

1) To foster creative day-dreaming.

2) To help participants clarify their core priorities and
   values.

3) To highlight the issues around the use and abuse of
   money in our culture.

GROUP SIZE

Any size group is appropriate.

TIME FRAME

20-30 minutes

MATERIALS NEEDED

A copy of the "Irish Sweepstakes" worksheet for each
participant.

PROCESS

1) The trainer announces that each participant has just
   won the million dollar Irish Sweepstakes. The check
   must be picked up in 20 minutes. The time until then
   will be spent planning what to do with the money.

2) The trainer provides each participant with an "Irish
   Sweepstakes" worksheet and guides everyone through
   the four questions, allowing ample time for participants
   to write their answers.

   ● Question #1, First Reactions: "What would you use
     the money for first? next? next?"

   ● Question #2, Budget Planning: Outline specific
     uses for all of the money; designate clear budget
     categories and allocations. When everyone is done,

ask what values this budget reflects.

*Note: The issue of personal values and priorities
        is obviously the key focus of this exercise.
        The more specific participants can be in
        writing their plans for use of the money,
        the more able they will be to examine the
        values and priorities expressed by their
        plans. Give people enough time to really
        work through and complete a budget.*

- Question #3, <u>Lifestyle Adjustments</u>: Imagine the
  changes that would take place in your life because
  of this bonanza.

- Question #4, <u>Reflections</u>: Examinine the values and
  priorities embedded in your responses to these
  questions.

3) The trainer divides participants into small discussion
   groups of four to six people each. Participants first
   share and compare their use of the money and the changes
   they imagine making in their lifestyle. Second, and
   most important, participants are to discuss the values
   and priorities they expressed in their budget alloca-
   tions, and describe the issues they struggled with
   while making the budget decisions.

4) In the closing plenary discussion the trainer may want
   to highlight the following themes:

- The variety of ways our culture uses, abuses and
  even worships money . . . and the effect of these
  dynamics on personal health.

- The importance of holding clear values and priorities, regardless of the amount of money we have.

- The issue of "spending for the present" vs "inves-
  ting for future security" which is more connected
  to personal style than it is to money. The way we
  use money is often only a mirror of how we spend
  ourselves -- our time and energy -- throughout
  life.

- Ask, "If a stranger looked at your answers, what
  would she conclude about your mission and purpose
  in life?"

THE IRISH SWEEPSTAKES

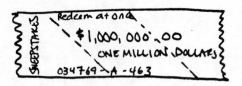

Here is your winning ticket for one million dollars in the
Irish Sweepstakes. You must redeem this ticket within 20
minutes. You will receive a check, cashable immediately.

1)   What will you do with the money?

   First I will _____ and then

   _____ and then _____

   _____ and then _____

   and then _____ and then _____

   _____ and then _____.

2)   Turn this paper over and make a tentative budget that
     accounts for what you would do with all of the money.
     (Include travel, books, recreation, new purchases,
     gifts/contributions, investments, savings, etc.) Make
     the budget total $1,000,000.

     After you have finished ask yourself what your budget
     tells you about your values.

3.   Reflect on the following questions:

■ How do you imagine you would want your life to change
  with such a nest egg?

  _____

■ What in your present lifestyle would you not want to
  have disrupted?

  _____

■ What dreams would you fulfill?

  _____

■ Would you continue to work at your present job?
  _____Why? or why not? _____

  _____

■ Having all the money you need --
    Why would you get up in the morning?

    _____

    When would you get up? _____
    What would you try to accomplish with your day?

    _____

4)   What do your answers tell you about yourself?

  _____
  _____
  _____

21 SPIRITUAL PILGRIMAGE

This lifeline drawing allows participants an opportunity to trace their spiritual journey, noting those experiences/ attitudes/revelations that contribute to their well-being and identifying areas for future growth.

GOALS

1) To raise consciousness about spiritual health as a component of well-being.

2) To affirm life experiences that have shaped participants' spiritual development.

GROUP SIZE

Unlimited; also appropriate for use with individuals.

TIME FRAME

20-30 minutes

MATERIALS NEEDED

A blank sheet of paper for each participant.

PROCESS

1) The trainer introduces the concept of spiritual health as an important dimension of whole person well-being, highlighting some or all of these points:

- Although we usually think of health in physical terms, health and wholeness are essentially spiritual concepts.

- Human beings are by nature spiritual -- we search for ultimate truth and purpose, we experience awe at the grandeur of creation, we forge our values in the crucible of life experience, we struggle with the questions of suffering and death, we accept the unknown on faith, we commit ourselves to causes and to service, we seek hope, faith and meaning in the face of despair. These are all signs of spiritual health.

- The human spirit can be a powerful healing force not only for life-threatening situations when restoration of health seems miraculous, but also for the day-to-day dis-eases we experience in all dimensions of life when relief sometimes seems no less miraculous.

- Each person has a unique spiritual heritage that contributes to his well-being and shapes his attitude toward self-care. Often people are not fully aware of the underlying spiritual issues that motivate their behavior.

2) Participants are instructed to use a blank sheet of paper to draw a timeline of their "spiritual pilgrimage" -- with all its ups and downs, twists and turns -- from birth up to the present.

The trainer suggests that they may want to include such events as a first encounter with death, times of clear (or clouded) purpose, values conflicts, awe-inspiring experiences, shifts in religious beliefs or practices, major commitments, significant rituals/celebrations, dry spells, difficult choices, moments of doubt.

Note: The trainer will need to allow plenty of time for participants to warm up to the drawing and will want to proceed slowly, suggesting different areas for consideration and giving examples to "prime the pump." Encourage participants to flesh out their drawings with labels or symbols that describe their journey.

3) Once participants have completed their past and present spiritual timelines, the trainer asks them to extend that line on into the future, predicting what spiritual growth lies ahead on their pilgrimage.

4) The trainer asks participants to reflect on their spiritual timeline and give themselves an overall grade for spiritual health. In deciding on the grade, people should note what two or three assets/qualities/experiences/attitudes raised the grade and which two or three lowered the grade.

5) Participants exchange timelines with someone else in their small group. After studying the diagrams for a few minutes, each person introduces her partner to the group by describing one or two qualities of his spiritual pilgrimage.

After these initial introductions, each group member describes her own spiritual lifeline in more detail. (15 minutes)

VARIATIONS

- If the group is small (12 or less), this exercise may be done as a whole group experience.

- The exchange of lifelines in Step #5 can be dropped. Participants introduce themselves, sharing as much of their spiritual pilgrimage as seems appropriate.

TRAINER'S NOTES

PLANNING

22. SHOULDS, WANTS, WILLS (p 97)

   A short planning exercise that invites participants to
   identify what they really want to do about their health
   and what action they are willing to take. (15-20 minutes)

23. WHAT DO YOU NEED? (p 100)

   This checklist helps participants identify qualities
   which may need personal attention/development.
   (10-15 minutes)

24. REAL TO IDEAL (p 104)

   In this simple planning exercise participants record their
   real and ideal health status in a variety of life areas
   then identify positive actions that could transform the
   real into the ideal. (10-15 minutes)

25. PERSONAL PRESCRIPTION (p 110)

   Participants write a personal prescription summarizing
   their self-care plan. (5-10 minutes)

26. MEET THE NEW ME (p 112)

   In this short closing ritual participants imagine the
   health and vitality they will possess one year later.
   They introduce themselves as if the positive changes they
   planned have already taken place. (10-15 minutes)

22 SHOULDS, WANTS, WILLS

In this short planning exercise, participants first identify the "shoulds" they have learned about self-care, then go on to discover what they really want to do about their health and what action they are willing to take.

GOALS

1) To help participants separate the "ought to's" from the "I really want to's" in self-care.

2) To elicit commitment to one or two clear self-care goals.

GROUP SIZE

Unlimited; may also be useful in work with individuals.

TIME FRAME

15-20 minutes

MATERIALS REQUIRED

A blank sheet of paper for each participant.

PROCESS

1) The trainer introduces the concept that people often pressure and overwhelm themselves with unrealistic or at least over optimistic expectations for change. It's not unusual for participants in a wellness course to be immobilized by the sheer number of changes they <u>could</u> make or "<u>should</u>" make in order to enhance their well-being. Not being able to follow through on all their good intentions, they accomplish none and feel frustrated and discouraged.

2) Participants are directed to take a piece of paper and fold it into thirds (like a letter). After opening the paper and turning it sideways they are asked to head the resulting three columns "SHOULDS" at the left, "WANTS" in the center and "WILLS" at the right.

3) The trainer asks participants to think back over the wellness training experience and list in the left hand column all the "SHOULDS" they have uncovered during the course (e.g. I should cut down my drinking,

start a support group, write to my mother, exercise
three times a week, etc) The trainer may want to
briefly review the topics or major points covered
during the course to help stimulate the participants'
memories.

4) When participants have stopped "shoulding" on themselves, they are asked to focus on the center section
of the worksheet. The trainer explains that what we
want to do is often lost in the morass of what we
think we should do. In the process we lose a prime
motivator and ally in the change process -- our natural
desire. Desire and motivation fade quickly as the
"agenda" for change lengthens.

Participants are invited to focus on what they truly
want to do in relation to self-care habits or lifestyle.

*Note: The trainer may want to reassure people that
at least some of them will probably not want
to do anything! That's fine. They are to be
absolutely clear about what they really want
to do about their health -- regardless of the
"shoulds."*

5) The trainer next asks participants to look over the
list of wants and shoulds and determine what self-
care actions they are willing to undertake during
the next month. The trainer invites people to write
their self-care commitments ("will do's") in the
right hand column. They are to list no more than
three! Of these three, no more than one may come
from the "SHOULD" column; at least two must come from
the "WANTS" column.

*Note: For persons who have no entries in the "WANT"
column, ask them to indicate what would transform each "should" into a "want" or "will."*

6) Participants may share their "WILL DO" plan with others
in their small group and, if desired, make a contract
with one or more group members to report back on the
success of their plan in one month.

Submitted by Gloria Singer

TRAINER'S NOTES

23 WHAT DO YOU NEED?

This checklist helps participants identify qualities which may need personal attention/development. This revealing exercise may be used as an independent icebreaker or assessment tool, but is especially effective near the end of a session.

GOALS

1) To identify personal needs/values.

2) To determine ways to meet those needs.

3) To see trends and categories of needs.

GROUP SIZE

Unlimited; also applicable for work with individuals.

TIME FRAME

10-15 minutes

MATERIALS NEEDED

A copy of the "What I Really Need" worksheet for each participant.

PROCESS

1) The trainer distributes the "What I Really Need" work-sheet and invites participants to complete Section A -- checking all words that would finish the sentence, "What I really need in my life right now is more . . ."

2) After everyone has finished the checklist the trainer may ask participants if they see any similarities in the items of each column (#1 physical, #2 mental/career, #3 emotional/relationships, #4 spiritual/self). The trainer may also ask people to notice any particular patterns in their present needs assessment.

3) The trainer then introduces Part B of the worksheet noting that participants will be able to develop many of their chosen qualities on their own, but for some they may need outside help. Participants are asked to underline the "do-it-yourself" needs and circle those that will require outside assistance.

As part of Step "B," participants should also identify people/institutions that might potentially help them meet the checked needs.

4) The trainer may ask participants to reflect on the balance between needs which the individual can develop alone and those qualities which the individual will want to seek help in developing. The trainer may challenge participants to reflect on which needs are most important -- and which ones they can start working on immediately.

5) The exercise concludes with a recommendation that participants save their worksheets and re-evaluate themselves in a few weeks, a few months or next year in order to check their progress and discover how their needs have changed.

VARIATIONS

- Participants may ask a spouse or close friend to fill out a duplicate questionnaire for them and then compare the two. "Do others see you as you see yourself?"

- Participants may share their discoveries with a partner or small group.

TRAINER'S NOTES

Submitted by Martha Belknap

WHAT I REALLY NEED IN MY LIFE RIGHT NOW IS MORE . . .

A. Check the words below which fit into this sentence for you. Add any other words which are also important in your life.

vitality	self-esteem	tenderness	composure
security	recognition	generosity	centering
activity	confidence	caring	awareness
health	motivation	sharing	solitude
strength	knowledge/skill	music	devotion
energy	opportunities	laughter	contemplation
fitness	challenges	support	serenity
relaxation	variety	self-expression	trust
comfort	structure	companionship	insight
nutrition	accomplishments	harmony	joy
touching	control	romance	commitment
sex	imagination	intimacy	communion
sleep	money	patience	integration
coordination	responsibility	beauty	forgiveness
flexibility	education/training	sensitivity	surrender
exercise	experience	receptivity	faith
self-control	freedom	self-awareness	purpose

B.   Study the qualities which you have checked. Underline the ones which you can develop
      by yourself. (Circle) the ones with which you will need some outside help. ✔ Check where
      you can receive the help you need.

         family

         friends

         partner/mate

         teacher/counselor

         doctor/nurse

         employer/employee/co-workers

         community center/church

         health facility/mental health center

         support group/club

         organization/institution

         school/university

24 REAL TO IDEAL

In this simple planning exercise participants record their real and ideal health status in a variety of life areas, then identify positive actions that could transform the real into the ideal.

GOALS

1) To identify health ideals.

2) To outline necessary steps for reaching health goals.

GROUP SIZE

Unlimited; could be used in work with individuals as well as groups.

TIME FRAME

10-15 minutes

MATERIALS NEEDED

"Real to Ideal" worksheet for all participants.

PROCESS

1) The trainer distributes the "Physical Real to Ideal" worksheets to all participants and asks them to record in the left hand boxes their current weight, blood pressure and cholesterol level (if known), then record their observations and assessment about actual alcohol, drug, tobacco, caffeine use, sleep patterns and tension management. People should describe as clearly as possible what is their REAL level, state or pattern.

2) The trainer then asks participants to reflect on what they believe would be the IDEAL weight, fitness level, sleep pattern, etc. and write that description of the "Ideal Me" in the corresponding right hand box.

3) Once everyone has completed this ideal self-portrait, the trainer points out the importance of positive visualization in attaining health goals, and starting with the first issue, weight, asks participants to visualize themselves actually reaching that ideal, asking questions like, "How do you feel?" "What steps did you take to reach this ideal"? "Who helped or

supported you?"   "What did you have to give up?"

After mentally responding to these questions, participants are directed to write in the middle column one
or more specific steps they could take to transform
their real health pattern into their ideal. They may
also make note of other people who could be supportive
to them in the process.

4) The trainer continues to guide participants through
the worksheet, moving to the next health concern and
asking people to visualize the real to ideal transfor-
mation process, until action steps have been identified
for each issue.

5) Participants are asked to look over the whole worksheet
and identify three specific steps they are willing to
take this week (or tomorrow) to start the transforma-
tion process.

6) If time and the group atmosphere allow, each person
may wish to stand up and declare one or more of his
resolutions for change.

VARIATIONS

- If the trainer prefers to focus on whole person health
transformations, the whole person "Real to Ideal" worksheet can be substituted. If time permits both the whole
person and physical worksheets may be utilized.

- Participants may be allowed to complete Step #4 at their
own pace rather than being led by the trainer.

TRAINER'S NOTES

REAL TO IDEAL WORKSHEET

	REAL	STEPS I COULD
WEIGHT		
BLOOD PRESSURE		
CHOLESTEROL LEVEL		
PHYSICAL FITNESS		
ALCOHOL USE		
DRUG USE (over the counter, RX)		
TOBACCO USE		
CAFFEINE USE		
SLEEP		
TENSION MANAGEMENT		

PHYSICAL

TAKE TO GET THERE	IDEAL

REAL TO IDEAL WORKSHEET

	REAL	STEPS TO
ENERGY LEVEL		
PHYSICAL SELF-CARE		
EMOTIONAL TONE & RANGE		
MENTAL SELF-CARE		
RELATIONSHIPS		
SELF-CONCEPT		
COMMITMENT		
CLARITY OF PURPOSE		

WHOLE PERSON

CHANGE	IDEAL

25 PERSONAL PRESCRIPTION

Participants write a personal prescription summarizing
their self-care plan. This brief exercise is best utilized
near the end of a course or workshop.

GOALS

1)   To reinforce plans for positive health habit change.

2)   To provide a reminder of self-care commitments.

GROUP SIZE

Unlimited; equally applicable for use with individuals.

TIME FRAME

5-10 minutes

MATERIALS NEEDED

A copy of the "Personal Prescription" form for each
participant.

PROCESS

*Note: This exercise must follow a more detailed self-care
        analysis and planning process.*

1)   The trainer distributes "Personal Prescription" forms
     to all participants and instructs them to summarize
     their self-care plan, being specific about how and
     when they plan to implement it.

     *Note: If people have difficulty filling out the Rx
             form, their plan is probably not clear and
             specific enough. The trainer may want to
             approach participants who have difficulty
             privately and offer consultation or structure
             an additional planning exercise for the entire
             group.*

2)   Once all have completed their prescriptions, the trainer
     directs participants to store them in their wallets and
     to take them out frequently as reminders of the goals
     they are trying to accomplish.

$R_\swarrow$

PERSONAL PRESCRIPTION

My Challenge to Myself

I, _____

would like to _____

and I will attempt to accomplish this in my life by

doing the following: _____ ,
                          (actions)

_____, _____,

and _____ which will be done by

_____.
    (frequency and date to be accomplished)

          Signed: _____

© 1983 Whole Person Press PO Box 3151 Duluth, MN 55803

26 MEET THE NEW ME!

In this short closing ritual participants imagine the
health and vitality they will possess one year later.
They introduce themselves as if the positive changes they
planned have already taken place.

GOALS

1) To help participants publicly affirm the goals they
   have set for themselves.

2) To provide a comfortable, positive way for participants
   to encourage each other and to wish each other well for
   the future.

GROUP SIZE

Any size group is appropriate; 10-15 participants per
group is optimal.

TIME FRAME

10-15 minutes

PROCESS

*Note: This exercise must follow the completion of some
lifestyle adjustment and goal setting planning process. In order for participants to introduce themselves as having successfully completed their plans,
they must have their goals and resolutions clearly
in mind.*

1) The trainer asks participants to write down the date
   one year from today. Then participants close their
   eyes and imagine it is one year later and they have
   successfully incorporated all their intended positive
   health behaviors into their life. The trainer slowly
   asks them a series of questions that focus on the
   fruits of their self-care improvements.

   □ What do you look like?
   □ What have you done that gives you pride?
   □ How are you feeling?
   □ How would you describe the "new" you?

   The trainer may ask participants to write down their
   answers in paragraph form, using the model below.

       _____(date). This year I have done _____
       _____, and _____, and _____
     and I feel _____, and _____, and ___
     _____. I am now _____.

2) The trainer forms participants into small groups, pre-
ferrably utilizing groupings that have shared together
earlier in the season/workshop. Groups stand in a
circle and face each other.

3) The trainer gives the following instructions:

> One at a time each person introduces herself <u>as if
> it were one year later</u> and <u>as if all positive self-
> care plans have been accomplished.</u>
>
> (e.g. "I want to introduce myself to you. Meet
> the new me! Last year I did _____, and
> _____, and _____ for myself
> and now I'm feeling _____.
>
> Everyone should declare this publicly one by one
> to the whole discussion group.
>
> The group members are encouraged to acknowledge
> and reinforce the fine achievement with cheers,
> applause, whistles, "amens," "congratulations," etc.

VARIATION

- The trainer may wish to instruct participants to introduce
themselves and brag about their improvement individually
with each person in their group. For this variation participants move to their right around the circle, touching
each person, introducing themselves, receiving the con-
gratulatory responses, then moving on to the next person.

  This format takes a bit longer but "forces" people to ver-
balize "the new me" more times, and allows participants
a chance to wish each other well on an individual basis.

TRAINER'S NOTES

ENERGIZERS

27 60-SECOND TENSION TAMERS

This exercise includes five brief techniques for letting go of tension, including deep breathing, stretches, shakes and TLT.

GOAL

1) To relax body tensions.

TIME FRAME

1 minute each

PROCESS

YAWN AND SIGH

1) The trainer asks participants to stand and take a big yawn or two, opening the mouth and throat until the "automatic yawn response" takes over. Encourage people to make noise as they yawn.

   Note: The trainer may want to demonstrate the yawn as she describes it, exaggerating the noise and action.

2) The trainer teaches people to sigh, demonstrating quiet inhale and the long noisy exhale that relaxes the throat and chest muscles. Participants practice noisy sighs.

3) The trainer leads the group in a sequence of yawn and sigh combinations.

STRETCH

1) The trainer instructs participants to stand and stretch -- arching their backs, stretching arms and fingers out wide, holding that position 5-10 seconds -- and then to let go, allowing their bodies to go completely limp.

2) Participants repeat this stretch two or three times.

SEDENTARY STRETCH

1) The trainer directs participants to sit up straight, bring their shoulders back as if trying to touch the blades together, hold that position for 7-8 seconds, and then release.

2) Next, participants are asked to curl their shoulders forward, as if trying to touch them in front, hold for 7-8 seconds, and release.

3) Participants repeat this "stretch for the sedentary" two or three times.

TRIPLE SHAKE

1) Participants stand with arms hanging loosely at their sides. The trainer asks them to shake their fingers, hands, wrists and arms on up to the shoulders. People should continue shaking until their arms feel warm and tingly. (10-20 seconds)

2) The trainer directs participants to use the same shaking procedure on their legs, one at a time. (10-20 seconds)

3) Finally, participants shake their trunk and whole body. (10-20 seconds)

TLT -- TENDER LOVING TOUCH

1) The trainer demonstrates the TLT -- Tender Loving Touch -- technique. He rubs his hands briskly together until they are warm, then lightly cups them over his closed eyes, with fingertips on the forehead, thumbs along the temple, heel of the hand on the cheeks.

2) Participants are instructed to warm their hands then cover their eyes in the TLT position. The trainer directs them to maintain this position for 2-3 minutes, letting go of all the tension in the eyes and face, and allowing themselves to slow down.

Submitted by Mary O'Brien Sippel

© 1983   Whole Person Press   PO Box 3151   Duluth, MN 55803

28 THE BIG MYTH

This stretching exercise asks participants to identify their "best" and then discover that often their "best" can really be bettered.

GOALS

1) To challenge the myth, "I'm doing the best I can."

2) To observe that often we underestimate our limits.

TIME FRAME

2 minutes

PROCESS

1) The trainer asks participants to stand and face the front of the room. With feet firmly planted about shoulder width apart and right arm outstretched, everyone should turn as far to the right as possible without straining.

2) The trainer directs people to notice the spot on the wall that represents their "best effort," making a mental note of where head and eyes are.

3) The trainer may gently challenge participants by asking, "Is this the best you can do? Your full capacity?" and noting that we often look at life issues and experience with the attitude -- "This is the best I can do, and I'll never be able to do any better." The trainer then suggests that such personal limitations can often be stretched and overcome.

4) Participants turn back to face the front of the room.

5) The trainer next directs everyone to turn their heads to the right again, while turning their eyes to the left; turn your body as far to the right as you can; then turn back to the front position.

6) This time participants turn head and eyes left; turn body to the right; turn back to the front.

7) Now everyone should turn head left and eyes right; turn body to the right as far as you can go; return to front position.

8) Finally, the trainer directs people to repeat Step #1,
    turning as far to the right as possible without strain-
    ing. The trainer asks, "Now how far did you go?" Most
    people will have turned a considerable distance further
    compared to the spot they had marked on the wall the
    first items.

9) The trainer may want to facilitate a group discussion
    about personal capabilities and how we're limited by our
    belief in the big myth -- "I'm doing the best I can."
    The trainer will want to reinforce the insight that we
    can easily surpass "best" efforts with a little stretch-
    ing and that everyone has within himself power to change.
    The discussion should touch on ways to raise personal
    "limits," to initiate more positive lifestyle changes
    and to not "accept things the way they are."

The exercise was submitted by Sandy Queen who first learned it
from Larry Wilson during the 1981 Wellness Strategies Workshop
at Stevens Point WI.

29 BREATHING MEDITATION

This centering activity combines regular breathing with mental affirmations.

GOALS

1) To center attention and quiet thoughts.

2) To reinforce positive health images.

TIME FRAME

1-2 minutes

PROCESS

1) The trainer instructs participants to close their eyes and mentally affirm statements to themselves as they breathe in and out.

2) The trainer describes the technique of affirming one phrase as they inhale and the companion phrase as they exhale.

3) The trainer reads the Centering Phrases one by one, pausing after each one to allow participants to repeat the words internally.

TRAINER'S NOTES

CENTERING PHRASES

<u>On the inhaling breath:</u>   <u>On the exhaling breath:</u>

I close my eyes . . . . and bring my awareness inside

I deepen my breathing . . . . . . and quiet my thoughts

I allow my body to be still . . . and relax my muscles

I focus into my center . . . . . and release my tensions
(frustration, anxiety,
fear, expectations)

I allow health to flow . . . . . and let go of disease
(pain, infection, fatigue,
discomfort, toxins)

I open my heart . . . . and free my spirit

I flow with life . . . . I am one with all

© 1983 Whole Person Press   PO Box 3151   Duluth, MN 55803

30 GRABWELL GROMMET

This humorous reading focuses on the "natural" consequences of negative self-care habits.

GOALS

1) To allow participants a chance to laugh at their own
    shortcomings.

TIME FRAME

5 minutes

PROCESS

1) The trainer reads the story, "It Was Just Natural."

It Was Just Natural

On the morning of his 42nd birthday, Grabwell Grommet
awoke to a peal of particularly ominous thunder. Glancing
out the window with bleary eyes, he saw written in fiery
letters across the sky: "Someone is trying to kill you,
Grabwell Grommet!"

With shaking hands Grommet lit his first cigarette of
the day. He didn't question the message. You don't
question a message like that. His only question was,
"Who?"

At breakfast, as he salted his fried eggs, he told his
wife, Gratia, "Someone's trying to kill me."

"Who?" she asked in horror.

Grommet slowly stirred the cream and sugar into his coffee
and shook his head. "I don't know," he said.

Convinced though he was, Grommet couldn't go to the police
with such a story. He decided that his only course was to
go about his daily routine and hope to somehow outwit his
would-be murderer.

He tried to think on his drive to the office. But the
frustration of making time by beating lights and switching
lanes occupied him wholly. Nor, once behind his desk
could he find a moment, what with jangling phones, urgent

memos and the problems and decisions piling up as they did every day.

It wasn't until his second martini at lunch that the full terror of his position struck him. It was all he could do to finish his lasagne milanese.

"I can't panic," he said to himself, lighting his cigar. "I simply must live my life as usual."

So he worked till seven as usual. Drove home fast as usual. Ate a hearty dinner as usual. Had his two cock-tails as usual. Studied business reports as usual. He took his usual two seconal capsules in order to get his usual six hours' sleep.

As the days passed he manfully stuck to his routine. And as the months went by, he began to take a perverse pleasure in his ability to survive. "Whoever's trying to get me," he'd say proudly to his wife, "hasn't got me yet. I'm too smart for him."

"Oh, please be careful," she'd reply, ladling him a second helping of beef stroganoff.

The pride grew as he managed to go on living for years. But, as it must to all men, death came at last to Grabwell Grommet. It came at his desk on a particularly busy day. He was 53.

His grief-stricken widow demanded a full autopsy.

But it showed only emphysema, arteriosclerosis, duodenal ulcers, cirrhosis of the liver, cardiac neurosis, a cerebravascular aneurism, pulmonary edema, obesity, cir-culatory insufficiency and a touch of cancer.

"How glad Grabwell would have been to know," said the widow, smiling proudly through her tears, "that he died of natural causes."

This story was distributed at a "summit conference" of the Minnesota Council on Health.

31 GROUP BACKRUB

Everyone joins in on this gigantic, simultaneous backrub.

GOALS

1) To provide tension release.

2) To promote contact among participants.

TIME FRAME

2-3 minutes

PROCESS

1) Without giving away the nature of this energizer the trainer asks the group to stand up, leave all their belongings at their seat, and move to form one huge circle around the room.

   Note: The larger the group, the more chaos this will cause and the longer it will take to form the circle. If possible, the circle should be single file. You may need to encourage the group to expand to include everyone or contract until a complete circle is formed. It is fine if the circle must cut between tables or chairs, or go around pillars, etc. Make sure everyone is close enough together to touch each other easily.

2) The trainer instructs everyone to turn to the right one quarter turn. Participants will now be facing the back of the person on their right. Participants move forward until they can put their hands on the shoulders of the person in front of them, and give that person a warm and relaxing backrub. Everyone in the circle will now be both giving and receiving a backrub simultaneously. The trainer encourages participants to massage the neck, arms and lower back, as well as the shoulders.

3) The trainer then instructs everyone to reverse directions and return the favor.

4) The trainer may briefly ask the participants what they notice about the change in their personal energy, as well as the total energy level in the room.

> *Note:* *Steps #1 and #2 must be distinctly separate. If*
> *the nature of the exercise is announced before*
> *the circle is formed, resisters -- who need the*
> *warmth of this exercise the most -- will end up*
> *watching from the edges of the room. When the*
> *circle is formed first, with no hints about*
> *what comes next, everyone will be "trapped"*
> *into participating and receiving the benefits.*

VARIATION

- Sometimes the size of the group, the nature of the room
  and the presence of tables, immovable chairs or other
  equipment makes the formation of a circle impossible. When
  this is true, the trainer skips the formation of a circle.
  Participants instead are asked to stand up, face the right
  wall, and move forward until they can massage the shoulders
  of the person in front of them. In this case, the massage
  is done in separate rows, with the front person only
  receiving, and the back person only giving a massage.
  Their turn comes, of course, when the direction is
  reversed.

32 MEGAPHONE

In this peppy exercise participants publicly acclaim
their personal wellness qualities.

GOAL

1)   To affirm personal health-enhancing qualities.

TIME FRAME

5-10 minutes

PROCESS

1)   The trainer asks participants to think of 2 personal
     qualities that enhance their health.

2)   The trainer instructs participants to choose one of
     the qualities and practice affirming it by whispering
     three times (as if to an imaginary friend) -- "I am
     _____." The trainer gives a signal and
     all participants whisper their individual health-full
     qualities at the same time.

3)   Next the trainer asks people to repeat their health-
     enhancing quality, saying it three times softly (as
     if to a lover). The trainer gives a signal and
     everyone speaks her quality together three times.

4)   This time the trainer suggests that at the signal
     participants affirm their qualities three times in
     a conversational tone (as if to a neighbor or someone
     in the carpool).

5)   The trainer now asks people to raise their voices (as
     if talking to a deaf uncle) and state the quality
     three times.

6)   Next the trainer directs participants to shout out
     loud (as if to a child upstairs).

7)   Finally, the trainer asks people to shout even louder
     (as if to a child upstairs with a stereo on). This
     is where the megaphone comes in!

8)   Repeat Steps #2-7 with the second quality. The trainer
     will need to keep the pace moving quite rapidly.

VARIATION

- In Step #1 the trainer may substitute affirmations that
  apply particularly to the session content (e.g. two qualities that you appreciate about yourself; two qualities
  that contribute to your emotional/spiritual/mental/
  relational health; two things you need; two qualities
  that make you a good friend, etc).

TRAINER'S NOTES

33 NOONTIME ENERGIZERS

This quick exercise encourages participants to tune into their own needs and to utilize the noontime break for revitalizing themselves and satisfying more than their hunger for food.

GOALS

1) To graphically demonstrate the opportunity for revitalization offered by the normal breaks built into the day.

2) To sensitize participants to the steady stream of needs they experience and to encourage them to respond creatively in ways that bring renewed vigor at the mid-day slump.

TIME FRAME

5-10 minutes

PROCESS

1) The trainer explains that we all have needs (hungers). These build up throughout the day and call for some satisfying responses on our part. If we don't respond, the needs become greater and we soon become fatigued. The trainer may want to describe need patterns in the following way:

> *Along with whatever else you've been doing all morning, you've been accumulating a variety of needs or hungers that are crying out for a response. Your stomach may want some food, your legs may need to stretch, etc. Not only does your body need replenishing, your soul may need to rest, too. You may be yearning for a meaningful conversation with someone of a like mind. You may just want to scream.*

> *If you respond to yourself and some of your non-dietary needs over the lunch hour, your stress will be diminished and you will experience a renewed sense of vitality with which to tackle the afternoon. If you instead charge on ahead through your "break," paying no attention to your internal signals during this noon hour, you'll face the afternoon even more tense and tired than you are*

now . . . and still hungry!

2) The trainer asks the group to close their eyes and listen to the variety of needs they are experiencing at this moment. The following questions, asked one at a time, at 30 second intervals, will guide participants in the process

   ☐ What is your body wanting right now? -- food, a stretch, a nap, exercise?

   ☐ What does your heart need right now? -- someone to appreciate you? quiet?

   ☐ What does your mind need right now? -- a chance to blank out? or sort out ideas? a new set of ideas?

   ☐ What do you need right now from other people? -- kindness? a smile? a chance to be alone? a hug? stimulation? support?

   ☐ What does your spirit need right now? -- centering? a chance to reflect? hope?

   The trainer comments, "You're probably in touch with quite a variety of needs (hungers) you're experiencing right now."

3) The trainer asks participants to keep their eyes closed and reflect over their own needs, considering how they could respond to as many as possible during the lunch hour.

   ☐ What could you do for your body? (Yes, besides eat!)

   ☐ How could you refill your heart?

   ☐ How could you give your mind what it needs?

   ☐ How could you use the lunch break to satisfy your need for people-contact or solitude?

   ☐ How could you nurture your spirit?

4) The trainer encourages participants to be clear and assertive in setting up their lunch hour to respond to as many of their needs as possible so that they may return in an hour with renewed energy, refreshed.

5) The trainer may distribute the "Noontime Energizers" worksheet as additional stimulation for participants.

6) After lunch and before beginning the next session the trainer may wish to ask the group for examples of

---

what they did and how well their plan worked. Often
the stories that emerge are delightful and stimulating.

The trainer may comment on the connection between such
self-nurture practices and vitality saying something
like, "You tell me what you do with your daily break
times, and I'll tell you which ones of you are bound to
burn out!"

VARIATION

- Obviously, this exercise may be utilized before a break
  at any time of the day, and is not confined to the lunch
  hour.

TRAINER'S NOTES

NOONTIME ENERGIZERS

Tune in to yourself and your lunch break needs.

- What do you need physically? What are your body's hungers right now?

- What do you need intellectually? What does your mind yearn for?

- What does your heart need? How is your self/other contact hunger?

- What does your spirit need?

TODAY make your lunch break a real break. Choose at least one imaginative and fun way of responding to your hungers. Here are a few ideas for starters. ENJOY!!

*read a book	*return to work 5 minutes
*meditate	early and do NOTHING
*eat breakfast food	*pick up litter
*organize your wallet	*take a nap
*take a cab somewhere	*write a letter
*get a hug	*smile at everyone
*compliment someone	*feed the pigeons
*see half a movie	*go to a museum
*look at the sky	*take a bus ride
*stretch every muscle	*visit a florist and breathe
*pretend you're blind	*call your mother (or lover)
*go in a closet and scream	*take five deep breaths
*buy something outrageous	*argue with someone
*ride every escalator	*listen to the city
*meet a stranger	*take a stranger to lunch

34 RED ROVER

Participants display their originality in moving from one side of the room to the other.

GOAL

1) To promote creative thinking and movement.

TIME FRAME

5-15 minutes depending on the size of the group.

PROCESS

1) The trainer asks everyone to stand and line up against the wall on one side of the room.

2) Participants are instructed to move one-by-one across the room to the opposite wall. After the first volunteer has crossed the room, the trainer divulges the rules of the game:

    ● Each person must cross the room differently from all the preceeding participants.

    ● The other participants watch the crossing and act as judges of originality. If any participant's style is not unique, she is sent back to try again.

3) Everyone crosses the room in turn until all have reached the opposite side.

    Note: Noise and laughter heighten the fun. The trainer may want to encourage coaching, cheering, jeering and applause.

VARIATION

■ If the class is large and the time is short, participants could move across the room in their small sharing groups, with each group crossing in a unique fashion.

Submitted by J J Cochran

35 SING ALONG

Everyone joins in a musical break that reinforces a wellness concept.

GOAL

1) To raise group spirit and affirm a whole person wellness attitude.

TIME FRAME

2-5 minutes

PROCESS

1) The trainer teaches the song "Silver and Gold" to participants, writing the words on a blackboard or newsprint poster:

> "Make new friends, but keep the old,
> One is silver and the other gold."

Note: If the trainer does not know this song, someone in the group probably will or ask a girl scout.

2) Once everyone has learned the tune and sung it in unison, the trainer divides the group into four sections. Section 1 starts the song, Section 2 comes in after the first phrase ("Make new friends"), then Section 3 followed by Section 4. Each section sings it through three times as a round.

VARIATION

- Substitute the calisthenics song, "Head, Shoulders, Knees and Toes" -- complete with all the pointing actions.

> "Head, shoulders, knees and toes, knees and toes;
> Head, shoulders, knees and toes, knees and toes;
> And eyes and ears and mouth and nose;
> Head, shoulders, knees and toes."

36 SLOGANS AND BUMPER STICKERS

Small groups of participants invent slogans that could be used for posters or bumper stickers in a wellness campaign.

GOALS

1) To reinforce wellness concepts and self-care strategies.

2) To spark creativity.

TIME FRAME

10-15 minutes

MATERIALS NEEDED

Newsprint and magic markers for each small group.

PROCESS

1) The trainer divides the participants into small groups (5-8 people).

2) Each group is given the task of creating catchy slogans that could be used on posters or bumper stickers for a wellness promotion campaign. (e.g. "Take Charge -- Stay Well" or "Conserve Energy -- Relax")

   Note: The trainer may want to narrow the focus some-what by assigning each group a target audience (kids, seniors, refugees, etc), a specific self-care behavior (relationship enhancement, chemical use, play, etc) or a particular well-ness concept (wholeness, spiritual health, self-responsibility, etc).

3) The groups spend 10 minutes inventing slogans, and writing them down on newsprint.

4) At the end of the brainstorming session, small group members choose their favorite slogan, make a sample poster or bumper sticker and present it to the group at large.

VARIATION

- With more time this exercise could be conducted as an inter-group competition. The trainer appoints a panel of judges to determine which group's slogan is best. The winning group members are treated to backrubs from the losers.

TRAINER'S NOTES

CONTRIBUTORS

Martha Belknap MA
Educational Consultant
395 Monroe
Denver CO 80206
303/321-0905 (home/office)

Martha is an educational consultant with a specialty in creative relaxation and stress
management skills. She has 25
years of teaching experience at
all levels. Martha offers
relaxation workshops and creativity courses through schools,
universities, hospitals and
businesses.

Thomas G Boman PhD
Professor, Dept of
   Professional Education
Univ of Minn, Duluth
Duluth MN 55812
218/726-7157 (campus)
218/724-2317 (off-campus)

Tom is a practicing educator,
in-service trainer and program
developer. Current interest in
the study of maintaining professional and personal high
vitality. Founder of the Society
for Orthosynergistic Behavior --
The Study of the Right Combina-
tion of Behaviors to Enhance
High Level Well-being. PhD in
Educational Psychology, MA in
Curriculum and Instruction,
BS in Chemistry.

J J Cochran
Partner/Trainer
The Icebreaker
4022 Pillsbury
Minneapolis MN 55409
612/831-4044 (office)

J J specializes in immediate
interactions of large groups
at conventions/seminars/meet-
ings/retreats to create an
atmosphere conducive to parti-
cipation, sharing of information,
and convention goals. Workshops/
seminars/speeches custom
designed on leadership, team
building, success, motivation,
self-esteem, communication,
leisure, appreciation.

Linda L Nowobielski
Educational Benefit Development
  Specialist-Personal Health
Aid Association for Lutherans
4321 Ballard Rd
Appleton WI   54919
414/734-5721 (office)

Linda received her BS in Community Health Education from
the University of Wisconsin-
La Crosse in 1978. Wellness
is a way of life for Linda,
both personally and profes-
sionally. Hobbies include
teaching the YMCA's aerobic
dance program, Fitness
Fantasia, weight training and
keeping current with the
health promotion field.

Sandy Queen
Director, Lifeworks
9 Folly Farms
Reisterstown MD   21136
301/526-6342 (office)

The author of Wellness for
Children and President-Elect
of the Organization of Wellness Networks, Sandy maintains
a busy practice as an independent health consultant. She
is best known in the Washington
area for her stress management
workshops in business and
industry. Sandy was recently
appointed to the Maryland
State Commission on Physical
Fitness.

Gloria Singer ACSW
Social Work Program Dir
College of St Scholastica
1200 Kenwood Ave
Duluth MN 55811
218/723-6129 (office)

Gloria is a social work educator with experience in teaching social policy, social work
methods and supervising field
instruction at the undergradu-
ate level. As a staff member
of the Gestalt Institute of
the Twin Cities she has also
taught in that organization's
Post-Graduate Training Program
in Gestalt Therapy. Her clini-
cal experience includes work
with individuals, couples and
groups.

Mary O'Brien Sippel, RN, MS
517 Lincoln Park Dr
Duluth MN 55806
218/722-8136 (home)
218/723-6130 (office)

Mary is still one of Whole Person Associates' most enthusiastic faculty. Now a counselor and faculty member at the College of St Scholastica, Mary continues to inspire others to care for themselves and stay vital. Mary's experience in teaching stress management across the country has enabled her to be her own best caretaker as career woman, wife and mother of two under two.

David X Swenson, PhD
Dir of Student Development
College of St Scholastica
1200 Kenwood Ave
Duluth MN 55811
218/724-6903 (home)
218/723-6085 (office)

A licensed psychologist, Dave maintains a private practice in addition to his administrative, educational and therapeutic roles at the college. He provides consultation and training to human services, health and law enforcement agencies.

THE EDITORS

All Handbook exercises not specifically documented are the creative efforts of the editors who have been designing, collecting and experimenting with structured processes in their teaching, training and consultation work since the late 1960's.

Nancy Loving Tubesing, EdD, holds a masters degree in group counseling and a doctorate in counselor education. She served as editor of the Society for Wholistic Medicine's monograph series and articulated the principles of whole person health care in the monograph, Philosophical Assumptions. A Faculty Associate and Publications Director at Whole Person Associates, Nancy is currently channeling her creativity and nearly boundless energy into the development of the Handbook series and the compilation and testing of exercises for future volumes.

Donald A Tubesing, MDiv, PhD, designer of the widely acclaimed STRESS SKILLS seminar and author of Kicking Your Stress Habits, has been a pioneer in the movement to reintegrate the body, mind and spirit in health care delivery. With his background in psychology, theology and education, Don brings the whole person perspective to his consultation in business and industry, government agencies and hundreds of health care and human service systems.

Both Nancy and Don have collaborated on many writing projects over the years, beginning with a small group college orientation project in 1970 and culminating in the publication of their new self-help book on whole person wellness, The Caring Question (Minneapolis: Augsburg, 1983).

FUTURE CONTRIBUTORS

If you develop an exciting, effective structured exercise you'd like to share with other trainers in the field of stress management or wellness promotion, please send it to us for consideration using the following guidelines:

1) Your entry should be written in a format similar to those in this Handbook.

2) Contributors must either guarantee that the materials they submit are not previously copyrighted or provide a copyright release for inclusion in the Whole Person Handbook series.

3) When you have adapted from the work of others, please acknowledge the original source of ideas or activities.

4) Include a brief (40 words) creative biography similar to those above.

All contributions will be acknowledged on receipt. The editors will review each submission and test it with one or more groups before reaching a decision about inclusion. Materials must be received by July 1st to be considered for the next years's Handbook volume. You will be notified by October 1st whether or not your exercise will be included.

© 1983   Whole Person Press   PO Box 3151   Duluth, MN 55803

WHOLE PERSON PUBLICATIONS

KICKING YOUR STRESS HABITS:
A do-it-yourself guide for coping with stress

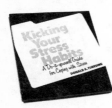

by Donald A Tubesing, MDiv, PhD

Striking graphics highlight this unusual "work-in-a-book" which actively engages the reader in in identifying sources of stress and resources for coping. Full of examples, worksheets, checklists, practical ideas and a planning process that really works! Ideal for classroom or group setting. Large format paperback, $10.00.

THE CARING QUESTION:
You first or me first -- choosing a healthy balance

by Donald A Tubesing & Nancy Loving Tubesing

Thought-provoking questions are scattered throughout this startling challenge to the wellness revolution. Filled with wit and wisdom, The Caring Question invites readers to move beyond wellness to a life that balances self-care with caring for others. Paperback, $3.75.

WHOLE PERSON HEALTH CARE: Philosophical Assumptions

by Nancy Loving Tubesing

This slim volume is packed with insights concerning the nature and form of whole person health care along with snapshots of the theory in practice, challenges to practitioners, and suggestions for research. Paperback, $6.00.

WHOLISTIC HEALTH:
A whole person approach to primary health care

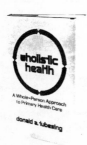

by Donald A Tubesing

This timely book calls for the redefinition of health and illness to include the whole person -- the mental, social, emotional and spiritual as well as the physical. Emphasizing an interdisciplinary approach to health education, early examination and prevention, it offers creative suggestions that can be applied by human service professionals in all settings. Hardcover, $19.95.

TAPE/WORKBOOK TRAINING PACKAGES

STRESS SKILLS: A structured strategy for helping people manage
                stress more effectively.

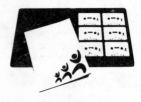

Voice-over narration guides the listener
through the celebrated STRESS SKILLS seminar
experience captured in these recordings.
Concept essays precede each worksheet in the
Participant Workbook and highlight topics
such as: the nature of stress, taking control of stress, choice and change, whole
person stress analysis and 20 stress skills.
Perfect for individual or small group study,
this resource would be a valuable addition
to any staff training library. Six cassettes
with companion workbook, $75.00. Workbook
only, $6.00.

TUNE IN: empathy training workshop

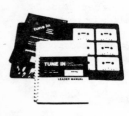

TUNE IN is a carefully developed and exten-
sively tested empathy training workshop you
can conduct yourself. The 16 hours of tape-
led group experiences help participants
develop competency in basic listening and
empathy skills. Currently used around the
world for inservice training of counselors,
teachers, physicians, hospital personnel,
volunteers, nurses, clergy, office staff,
managers and administrators. Workshop
tapes, Leader Manual and Participant Workbook, $75.00. Workbook only, $6.00.

R$_x$ for BURNOUT: Promoting vitality and preventing burnout in the
                  care-giving professions.

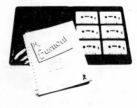

Carefully edited, attractively packaged
cassette recordings of a live, R$_x$ for BURNOUT
workshop can be used with the accompanying
Participant Workbook to create the seminar
atmosphere and process. Topics include:
symptoms, stages and causes, stress/vitality
in the workplace, individual revitalization
strategies, interpersonal support networking
and planning for renewal. Order this pack-
age for conducting your own workshop or to
share with friends and colleagues. Tapes and
workbooks, $75.00. Workbook only, $6.00.

CASSETTE TAPES

RELAX . . . LET GO . . . RELAX

> This unusual cassette offers the listener both a 30-minute
> "end of the day" relaxation experience for shedding ten-
> sion and a 20-minute "any time of the day" revitalization
> routine for p.r.n. refreshment. Male and female narration.
> Cassette in holder, $7.50.

> *HALPERN SOUND SETTING*

> *RELAX . . . LET GO . . . RELAX is now available with
> soothing musical background by Steven Halpern, PhD. This
> revolutionary "anti-frantic alternative" music is specifi-
> cally designed to trigger a deep state of relaxation and
> promote physical and mental well-being. Tape in holder,
> $9.00.*

SPIRITUAL CENTERING: An inward journey of renewal

> In this non-judgmental exploration of personal spiritual
> depths, Don Tubesing guides listeners through a process
> of quieting and centering that allows each person to dis-
> cover her own internal wisdom. A deep and moving experience
> that produces feelings of love and acceptance. Useful as a
> discussion starter or closing motivator. Flip side with
> Halpern Sounds musical background. Tape in holder, $9.00.

FINGERTIP FACE MASSAGE

> In her warm and gentle manner, Mary O'Brien Sippel guides
> listeners through a non-threatening self-massage process.
> The experience generates a feeling of relaxation, well-
> being and renewed vitality. Use this tape as an "energy
> break" during long sessions or to kick off your presenta-
> tion of self-care options. Flip side with Halpern Sounds
> musical background. Tape in holder, $9.00.

YOU ALONE CAN BE WELL . . . BUT YOU CAN'T BE WELL ALONE!

> In this keynote speech from Wellness Promo VII, Dr Donald
> Tubesing addresses the issue of wellness from the whole
> person perspective, asking the question, "What's the
> point of being well?" Listeners are asked to reflect on
> the self/other care balance in their lives. A humorous,
> challenging, positive 90 minutes. Tape in holder, $7.50.

THE WHOLE PERSON HANDBOOK SERIES
FOR TRAINERS, EDUCATORS, AND GROUP LEADERS

STRUCTURED EXERCISES IN STRESS MANAGEMENT   VOLUME I

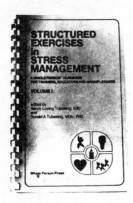

Nancy Loving Tubesing, EdD and
Donald A Tubesing, PhD, Editors

36 ready-to-use teaching designs that
involve the participant as a whole person
in learning to manage stress more effec-
tively. These exercises help motivate
participants to identify desired changes,
build new coping skills and plan for a
healthier lifestyle.

Includes icebreakers, assessments, theme
expanders, skill builders, action planners
and group energizers. Spiral bound,
flexible plastic cover, $12.50.

STRUCTURED EXERCISES IN WELLNESS PROMOTION   VOLUME I

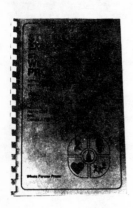

Nancy Loving Tubesing, EdD and
Donald A Tubesing, PhD, Editors

36 experiential learning activities that
focus on whole person health -- body,
mind, spirit, emotions, relationships.
These exercises encourage people to adopt
a wellness-oriented attitude and develop
more responsible self-care patterns.

Includes icebreakers, wellness explora-
tions, self-care strategies, action
planners and group energizers. Spiral
bound, soft plastic cover, $12.50.

© 1983 Whole Person Press   PO Box 3151   Duluth, MN 55803

ORDER FORM

SHIP BY RETURN MAIL TO:

Name _____

Address _____

_____

City _____

State _____ Zip _____

PO # _____

Please make checks payable and
send to:
Whole Person Associates Inc
2525 E 2nd St
PO Box 3151
Duluth MN 55803
218/728-4077

PLEASE SEND:

	price	total
WHOLE PERSON HANDBOOKS		
FOR TRAINERS, EDUCATORS & GROUP LEADERS		
☐ Structured Exercises in Stress Management (I)	$12.50	_____
☐ Structured Exercises in Wellness Promotion (I)	12.50	_____
TAPE/WORKBOOK TRAINING PACKAGES		
☐ STRESS SKILLS workshop	75.00	_____
☐ TUNE IN workshop	75.00	_____
☐ Rx for BURNOUT workshop	75.00	_____
WORKBOOKS ONLY		
☐ STRESS SKILLS Participant Workbook	6.00	_____
☐ TUNE IN Participant Workbook	6.00	_____
☐ Rx for BURNOUT Participant Workbook	6.00	_____
BOOKS		
☐ Kicking Your Stress Habits	10.00	_____
☐ The Caring Question	3.75	_____
☐ Philosophical Assumptions	6.00	_____
☐ Wholistic Health	19.95	_____
TAPES		
☐ Relax . . . Let Go . . . Relax	7.50	_____
☐ Relax (with Halpern Sounds)	9.00	_____
☐ Spiritual Centering	9.00	_____
☐ Fingertip Face Massage	9.00	_____
☐ You Alone Can Be Well . . . But You Can't		
Be Well Alone!	7.50	_____

HOW TO ORDER

As a small publisher we appreciate your interest
in our publications. We fill orders promptly when
the guidelines below are followed.
Terms. Orders from individuals must be accompanied by payment in full. Institutional purchase
orders must accompany requests for purchases on
credit. Net 30 days.
Shipping and handling. Please add $1.50 for
the first item and 50¢ for each additional item to
cover shipping and handling.

SUBTOTAL _____

(TAX—MN 5%) _____

SHIPPING _____

GRAND TOTAL _____